Antonio Colombo   Goran S

Colombo's
Tips
& Tricks
in Interventional Cardiology

MARTIN DUNITZ

Colombo's Tips and Tricks in Interventional Cardiology

Colombo's Tips and Tricks in Interventional Cardiology

Antonio Colombo, MD

Director, Cardiac Catheterization Laboratory
EMO Centro Cuore Columbus
Director, Cardiac Catheterization Laboratory and Interventional
Cardiology
San Raffaele Hospital
Milan, Italy
Director of Investigational Angioplasty
Lenox Hill Hospital
New York NY,
USA

Goran Stankovic, MD

Research Coordinator
EMO Centro Cuore Columbus and San Raffaele Hospital
Milan, Italy

MARTIN DUNITZ

First published in the United Kingdom in 2002
by Martin Dunitz Ltd, The Livery House, 7–9 Pratt Street, London NW1 0AE

Tel.: +44 (0) 20 7482 2202
Fax.: +44 (0) 20 7267 0159
E-mail: info.dunitz@tandf.co.uk
Website: http://www.dunitz.co.uk

Although every effort has been made to ensure that drug doses and other information are
presented accurately in this publication, the ultimate responsibility rests with the
prescribing physician. Neither the publishers nor the authors can be held responsible for
errors or for any consequences arising from the use of information contained herein. For
detailed prescribing information or instructions on the use of any product or procedure
discussed herein, please consult the prescribing information or instructional material
issued by the manufacturer.

A CIP record for this book is available from the British Library.

ISBN 1 84184 125 0

Distributed in the USA by
Fulfilment Center
Taylor & Francis
7625 Empire Drive
Florence, KY 41042, USA
Toll Free Tel: 1–800–634–7064
E-mail: cserve@routledge_ny.com

Distributed in Canada by
Taylor & Francis
74 Rolark Drive
Scarborough
Ontario M1R 4G2, Canada
Toll Free Tel: 1–877–226–2237
E-mail: tal_fran@istar.ca

Distributed in the rest of the world by
ITPS Limited
Cheriton House
North Way, Andover
Hampshire SP10 5BE, UK
Tel: +44 (0)1264 332424
E-mail: reception@itps.co.uk

Printed and bound in Great Britain

Contents

Preface

Antonio Colombo's *Tips and Tricks* attempts to summarize in a few sessions a number of practical concepts that, with practice, have guided and advanced the skills of an interventional cardiologist through 15 years in the cath lab.

The objective is to convey practical points frequently not discussed in formal presentations. The material and the approach presented on these CD-ROMs are not always what could be defined as 'standard practice': they are the opinionated view of one person. This fact makes the program unique. As I said to the audience at the beginning of the Paris Course on Revascularization 2001 session: "It is the first time for me to structure this type of format."

The topics covered are areas I consider most relevant in our field of interventional cardiology and which are frequently not discussed completely in many presentations. It is important to say that we skipped areas already well covered in many other presentations. If a topic has not been discussed, this does not mean it is not relevant.

When this entire job was completed, we decided to organize all the material into a book mainly based on visual presentations. The written part is limited to the essential comments to guide the reader through the four CDs. There are two additional chapters on stent selection and on pharmacology to prevent restenosis that we felt important to include.

Major thanks and recognitions should go to Professor Jean Marco and to all the Directors of the EuroPCR who had the idea to include this program in one of the most important events in interventional cardiology. Without their visionary planning, all this work would not exist. Thanks to all the Faculty Members of Tips and Tricks who contributed during the meeting with their presentations and very diligently edited the material for this book.

Dr. Goran Stankovic needs a special recognition for devoting six months of his time and his superb skills to put together into structured case presentations my ideas.

Thanks also to Alan Burgess, our commissioning editor at Martin Dunitz Ltd, whose goal has always been to publish the best in interventional cardiology.

Above all, we need to thank the 'wine', as Professor Giancarlo Biamino told me that the idea of *Tips and Tricks* came during a meeting of the Directors of the EuroPCR only after the second bottle of a good French red wine.

Antonio Colombo
Milan, New York

Background and Case Summaries

Disk 1

1 General approach

Introduction

The first thing that comes to our minds is that with cardiovascular interventions made so easy and, in most situations, predictable, it is very difficult to propose using anything but a stent. TA Bass recently wrote:

> "Through the years I've come to respect the importance of simplicity, any procedure or modification that add complexity, risk or cost need to be carefully scrutinized and might demonstrate very clearly that there is a benefit"
>
> (*Cathet Cardiovasc Interven* 2001; **53**; 21–22).

These allusions are made toward intravascular ultrasound (IVUS), atherectomy, thrombus aspiration, and many new devices that confront us almost daily.

In these first few slides I have tried to show you that in a number of selected cases, we require something more than a simple stent.

The results of the two largest randomized trials of stenting versus surgery, Arterial Revascularization Therapy Study (Arts) and Stent or Surgery Trial (SOS), are acceptable and superior compared to percutaneous transluminal coronary angioplasty (PTCA), but still not so good as to make a number of cardiologists advocates of interventional procedures.

One of the major problems with stenting is its user-friendly characteristics that make this device suitable for any type of lesion. The temptation to rebuild the coronary tree is quite high. In addition, the current new generation stents give such a nice and smooth angiographic result that the need to improve the result by further expanding the stent becomes less and less evident.

My general approach is: if you have a simple anatomy, a simple lesion and a relative simple clinical setting, just do simple stenting. There is no reason whatsoever to complicate what is not complicated to start. If the clinical scenario is not so simple, you may need to resort to a more

3

complex procedure. What I mean by simple or complex is not just the anatomy of the patient or the characteristics of the lesion, it is also the clinical context associated with the risk of restenosis.

Approach to ostial lesions

DCA for ostial LAD

Case 1

I want to commence discussion of the above-mentioned issues with a typical situation such as an ostial left anterior descending (LAD) lesion. This is the type of lesion that can be treated with a left internal mammary artery (LIMA) with a very good long-term outcome.

> When dealing with an ostial or very proximal LAD, if you want to compete effectively with surgery, you need to offer more than a 20%–30% risk reduction of restenosis.

The one reason to keep directional atherectomy (DCA) alive is this one. We say this because our data support that DCA and stenting are associated with a better long-term outcome. Yet, if this is the case, why not propose DCA and stenting for most of the lesions?

> We need to go back to the original statement: make the procedure more complex when it is really necessary or when the gain for an improved outcome is important. In addition, it is necessary to take into account the technical difficulties and risks to perform DCA in a proximal LAD lesion versus many other coronary lesions in locations more difficult to reach.

At the present time with the Flexicut DCA device (Guidant, Temecula, CA), the procedure is friendlier for both the operator and the patient.

The only guidewire we recommend with the Flexicut is the Ironman (Guidant, Temecula, CA), and for very difficult cases, the Platinum Plus (Boston Scientific, Maple Grove, MN). The Platinum Plus needs to be used as a second wire and exchanged following lesion crossing with a more delicate wire. The Ironman can be used as a primary wire in some lesions, but do not try to use it always as the primary wire. If the anatomy is complex or you are not sure perform a wire exchange. The lesion presented here can be crossed directly with the Ironman wire.

Then, we performed DCA and implanted a stent. This is one approach to the ostial lesion that we consider the best for very proximal LAD stenosis.

Where are the data? We have no hard clinical data, only data coming from registries.

We need to wait for the results of the Atherectomy before Multi-Link Improves Gain and Clinical Outcomes (AMIGO) trial, and we hope the investigators performed good DCA. We should remember that debulking does not work simply because we intend to do it!

Stent versus stent plus

Case 2

A possible alternative to the DCA-and-stent approach for ostial lesions is to use a cutting balloon and stents.

> I like to call the cutting balloon 'the simple atherectomy device, the poor man's atherectomy device.' We admit that this second approach is supported only by theoretical data and no large registry data are at present available.

If you decide to perform interventions with a cutting balloon prior to stenting, IVUS may be useful to size the cutting balloon appropriately. You should not feel upset or believe you did a bad job if this strategy produces a dissection that requires a longer stent. Full dilatation of a lesion may sometimes produce a dissection. It is important to keep this in mind: when you size the cutting balloon by IVUS you should round off to the lower quarter-size just for safety.

This vessel measured 4mm by IVUS; therefore, a cutting balloon of 3.75mm appears a reasonable choice.

The fact you see a dissection after using a cutting balloon is not unexpected: you cut, so you might see some dissection; you are going to stent anyway, so there is no reason to be worried!

In this case, we did something more than just place a stent. We placed a drug-eluting stent that is still an investigational device: the Quanam sleeve taxol-derivate drug-covered stent (Quanam Medical Corporation, Santa Clara, CA).

Following stenting, you see a frequent side-effect: a new narrowing now present at the ostium of the circumflex. Unfortunately, this side-effect is not rare.

What you do at this point? Often, it is just spasm treatable with intracoronary nitroglycerin. In this case we performed IVUS in an attempt to learn more. This test is not sufficient to rule out spasm, because you can have spasm around the IVUS catheter that looks like narrowing. If you are a good observer, you will notice narrowing without much plaque.

Finally, we used low pressure inflation with a 2.5mm balloon to achieve a good final angiographic result. The result was not satisfactory; we finally stented the ostium of the circumflex. Good luck for preventing restenosis!

The follow-up angiogram highlights several problems: despite an excellent lumen inside the Quanam stent there is a stenosis in the distal end of the stent; this is probably caused by trauma of the protruding balloon; the stent at the level of the circumflex shows in-stent restenosis which is not an unusual problem for standard stainless steel stents.

For me, the message is that you have to resist placing a second stent if the lesion, at the beginning, was not critical. If there is clear plaque shift or a dissection, the story is different. To implant a second stent is not always best for the patient.

If you are not satisfied by finishing with an intermediate result, do a 'massage' with an undersized balloon without dissecting, just to get a reasonable final result.

At the time of treatment of this restenosis, we placed a second stent distally to the Quanam stent and used a cutting balloon on the stent restenosis of the circumflex.

Dissections

These cases are presented to highlight the problem of dissections.

> Despite the current equation which states dissection = stent, an interventionist needs to know:
>
> - when he can leave a dissection without a stent,
> - when it is necessary to make this consideration,
> - what are the tools you use to make the final decision.

In general we agree with the current teaching that most dissections need stenting, and this attitude is the safest conduct for the patient and for the operator. Still, there are conditions in which it is better not to stent or in which it may not be possible to place a stent: these types of situation are frequently difficult and potentially more dangerous and risky compared to leaving the dissection. It must be understood that all this reasoning is based on the fact we have tools to differentiate a 'benign' dissection, one which can be left as such because the probability of it closing is low, versus a malignant dissection which may close.

> It is not acceptable to leave a dissection basing your decision on the angiographic appearance or on a vague feeling that there are good chances the dissection will stay open.

Case 3

This patient has a lesion on a protected left main coronary artery that involves a trifurcation with the proximal LAD, an intermediate branch and the circumflex.

The LIMA was implanted quite distally. It is important in this case to maintain patency of the proximal LAD stump. Following predilatation, a large dissection involving the three branches becomes evident.

Even a very experienced operator may have difficulty in deciding which way to stent appropriately this dissection involving three vessels. The fact that there is no flow impairment toward any of the branches is an important point to take into consideration.

The next step is to evaluate if this dissection is flow-limiting or not, and if there is any possibility to leave it as such. To make this decision, we use the pressure gradient, measured with a multifunction probing catheter, across the dissection. This catheter is a dual-lumen monorail catheter (Boston Scientific, Maple Grove, MN). The monorail lumen is used to advance the catheter over the wire already in place. The coaxial lumen serves to measure the distal pressure. The catheter is 3F, and the absence of a significant gradient (<20mmHg) is reassuring. It is worth mentioning that the multifunctional probing catheter can also be used for other purposes, such as evaluation of the distal flow with a selective injection (to distinguish between a mechanical obstruction and a failure of the microcirculation), distal injection of various drugs, and wire exchange.

In this specific case, the pull-back gradient was 15mmHg. This finding is sufficient to confirm that this specific dissection will stay open. There is literature from the earliest times of coronary angioplasty supporting the value of a low (<20mmHg) resting gradient across a dissection as an important element to predict lesion patency at follow-up.

The next cine run was obtained three days later. There was no stenting. We lost some branches in the dissecting process, but all the main vessels were open with good distal flow – it is difficult to believe that these branches would have stayed open following extensive stenting. This patient was left as such. He had a non-Q-wave myocardial infarction (MI) and has been asymptomatic throughout a six-month follow-up period. The follow-up angiography revealed good patency of the dissected segments, with complete healing of the dissection. In one segment of the obtuse marginal branch, there was a focal stenosis which was easily treated by stenting.

Case 4

This is an example of a long lesion of the LAD. The lesion was initially treated with balloon angioplasty, followed by atherectomy and stenting. A dissection is present distal to the stent. This dissection was left as such following evaluation of the residual lumen by IVUS.

We limited the treatment to one stent. What is the value or the risk of placing another stent? It depends which school of thought you embrace. If you believe that long stents create more restenosis, then that is a sufficient reason to place a second stent. We looked at long-term outcomes in patients left with a dissection. The outcomes in terms of events and restenosis were not different from a matched group without dissections.

Reopening an occluded SVG

Let us now switch the topic to totally-occluded vein grafts. The general attitude is to leave occluded grafts the way they are.

Case 5

The patient we present here had surgery performed a few days before this angiogram. The patient developed severe heart failure with ECG changes compatible with ischemia; this is the reason why the angiogram and the attempt to reopen the graft were performed.

The occluded graft was reopened with a Choice PT wire (Boston Scientific, Maple Grove, MN), the thrombotic material was removed with the Angiojet device (Possis Medical, Minneapolis, MN) and stenting was performed. When these types of interventions are performed, we need to keep in mind the danger of distal embolization.

It is no longer acceptable to use simple balloon angioplasty or direct stenting to treat these occlusions. A thrombus removal device and possibly a distal protection device must be used in order to avoid massive distal embolization.

Treatment of slow flow

Other devices that could be used are the X-Sizer atherectomy or rather thrombectomy catheter (Endicor Medical, Valkenswaard, The Netherlands) or the Rescue thrombus aspiration catheter (Boston Scientific, Maple Grove, MN).

In the event the patient develops slow flow, the best approach, in our view, is to use sodium nitroprusside 40μg bolus into the graft.

Case 6

This case illustrates current treatment of slow flow.

Shown is a distal right coronary artery with in-stent restenosis. The lesion was treated with a cutting balloon, with the occurrence of severe slow flow. In our experience, it is quite rare to see such severe slow flow in the setting of in-stent restenosis.

As we said, the treatment consisted of selective injection of 40–80µg of sodium nitroprusside. A clear improvement is demonstrated in the angiogram, obtained after a few seconds. At the present time, this pharmacological approach replaces adenosine or calcium channel blockers for the treatment of slow flow.

Preparation of the sodium nitroprusside infusion is as follows: one ampoule of nypride which equals 100mg is diluted with 250ml of 5% glucose solution; with a 20ml syringe you take 1ml of this solution (400µg of nypride) and dilute with 19ml of 5% glucose. The final solution will contain 20µg of nypride per ml. Usually, you will administer 3–4ml at a time.

Test for endothelial dysfunction

Case 7
This case demonstrates the evaluation of a patient affected by severe angina in which a coronary angiogram showed normal coronary arteries. Possible diagnoses include endothelial dysfunction.

This diagnosis is made by excluding microcirculatory disease (intracoronary Doppler with normal coronary flow reserve [CFR]), by excluding coronary atherosclerosis (normal IVUS), and by demonstrating a paradoxical vasoconstriction following intracoronary infusion of acetylcholine

Quanam stent for restenosis

Case 8
This patient had recurrent restenosis. He underwent five angioplasties, including one procedure with brachytherapy on his protected left main coronary artery. The procedure presented here is the implantation of a Quanam sleeve taxol-derivate drug covered stent (Quanam Medical Corporation, Santa Clara, CA), placed at the ostium of the LAD. Following implantation of the stent on the LAD, there is a worsening of a non-significant lesion present on the circumflex.

This new lesion was treated with a 2.5mm balloon inflated at low pressure.

Complications with new therapeutical approaches: PTCA failure, no brachytherapy failure

Case 9

This is a case of brachytherapy failure, which in reality may be better called angioplasty failure.

The analysis of the dilatation procedure of the restenotic lesion inside the stented segment, performed prior to brachytherapy, shows that in the short segment between the stents the dilating balloon does not fully expand. The IVUS study shows a persistent luminal narrowing, which is evaluated as not critical by angiography. The radiation therapy was performed with gamma radiation, using a 10-seed catheter and delivering 14Gy at 2mm depth. The follow-up angiogram shows a severe stenosis occurring at the site of the original suboptimal PTCA result.

> This case illustrates how important it is to obtain an acceptable angiographic result prior to brachytherapy; moreover, it also shows that in many situations this optimal result may be quite difficult to obtain, especially if the operator tries to avoid stenting the lesion.

Complications with new therapeutical approaches

Brachytherapy late thrombosis 1 & 2

Cases 10 and 11

These cases present one rare but devastating problem: late stent thrombosis following intracoronary brachytherapy. In both patients, this complication occurred at 1 year following brachytherapy. The patients discontinued ticlopidine therapy and were taking only aspirin. The problem of dependency on double antiplatelet therapy following brachytherapy and stenting is not trivial. Even if the patient tolerates this therapy well, it is not rare that other events, such as various types of surgery (e.g. prostatectomy, biopsy, etc.), may demand temporary discontinuation of ticlopidine. This situation places the doctor and the patient under a significant amount of stress and uncertainty.

Drug stent thrombosis

The sleeve drug-coated stent (Quanam stent) is not free from the above risk.

Case 12
This case illustrates drug stent thrombosis. Following reopening of a chronic total occlusion (CTO) of the LAD, a Quanam sleeve drug-coated stent was implanted at the site of the occlusion.

The 7-month angiographic follow-up showed optimal patency of the stented site. Following the diagnostic angiogram, according to the study protocol, the patient was advised to stop ticlopidine and continue with aspirin only. Two weeks later the patient sustained an MI and a new angiogram demonstrated complete occlusion of the LAD at the stented site.

Hopefully, the drug-coated stents without a polymer sleeve will not be associated with this risk of late thrombosis.

Complications with new therapeutical approaches: Primum non nocere

Case 13
This case illustrates the failure of a modern therapy aimed at prevention of restenosis and the related side-effects. The patient had a focal mid-LAD stenosis which was treated with stent implantation and then underwent, as part of a research protocol, beta-radiation brachytherapy. The follow-up angiogram shows patency of the stented segment and a severe proximal and distal stenosis. This pattern of restenosis has been called 'candy wrapper' and it has been associated with the implantation of radioactive stents. The specific problem in this case is that, for reasons not yet clear, this patient underwent three recurrences requiring a total of four procedures to treat what was initially a focal LAD stenosis. Certainly, the brachytherapy triggered an aggressive proliferation which became difficult to manage.

> These few cases were included to raise our attention toward the rare but quite devastating complications sometimes associated with new therapeutical modalities such as radiation therapy or drug-coated stents.

2 My first stent thrombosis

Case 14

This case belongs to history: we are in 1989. It is our first case of stent thrombosis.

The patient had a Palmaz–Schatz stent placed in the proximal LAD to treat a PTCA restenosis. A few days following stenting, while still on heparin infusion and waiting to reach an appropriate value of anticoagulation with coumadin, the patient sustained stent thrombosis.

The interesting aspects of this case are summarized In the letter written by Richard Schatz.

The importance of antiplatelet therapy (at that time credit was given to persantine) and of stent optimal dilatation is well-emphasized, a visionary perception about the future of coronary stenting.

3 Complications

Aortic dissections during PCI

Cases 15–18

The first set of complications presented here are dissections of the aortic wall caused by the tip of the guiding catheter. These types of complications are more common during procedures performed on the right coronary artery (RCA).

> Our attitude toward these dissections is to do our utmost to maintain a conservative management. It is important to exclude the presence of aortic regurgitation, dissections involving the supraaortic vessels, and progression of the original dissection. If none of these problems is present, a watchful waiting is the best attitude.

Right internal mammary artery (RIMA) dissection

Case 19

We observed an extensive dissection starting at the ostium of a mammary artery grafted to the LAD. The salient aspect of this case is that the dissection was not detected, because filming was not performed with the guiding catheter partially disengaged from the ostium. The patient experienced severe ischemia a few minutes after the end of the procedure. A new angiogram revealed an extensive dissection of the mammary artery beginning at the ostium. Extensive stenting of the entire mammary artery was performed to establish patency and normal flow. Despite the implantation of many long stents, covering the entire mammary artery, the patient developed only focal restenosis that was treated with repeat angioplasty.

Cutting balloon trapped in a stent

Case 20

The case describes a rare but problematic complication: entrapment of a cutting balloon in an NIR stent (Medinol/Boston Scientific, Maple Grove, MN) positioned at the ostium of the circumflex artery. In this particular case, the cutting balloon did not traverse the stent struts to dilate a side branch, a situation seen by the operator as risky for potential balloon entrapment. The cutting balloon was positioned inside the stent, which was implanted at the ostium of the circumflex artery. The balloon inflated and deflated well, but could not be pulled back from the stent. Despite a number of maneuvers, including attempts to negotiate another balloon alongside the trapped balloon, the balloon could not be removed and the patient was referred for emergency surgery.

The following lessons can be learned from this adverse event:

- A cutting balloon should be only advanced to half of its length through the stent struts (balloons should never be advanced completely).
- Advancement into the side branch should be avoided if the angle between the origin of the branch and the main vessel is close to or more than 90°.
- The cutting balloon should not be used when the stent to be crossed into the side branch is a closed-cell stent such as the NIR stent.
- If the operator has doubts it is better to use a regular balloon.

PTCA without heparin

Case 21

Case 21 illustrates a complication which can be called: 'Do not introduce any diagnostic or therapeutic device into the coronary arteries unless the patient has been anticoagulated with heparin.'

The patient was referred for a diagnostic angiogram and possible angioplasty because of post-infarction angina. The patient sustained an MI. An echocardiogram raised the suspicion of possible hemopericardium with a contained rupture. The diagnostic angiogram showed an occlusion of the circumflex coronary artery. The operator felt that a recent occlusion with a favorable anatomy could be easily and quickly (two words that should not exist in the vocabulary of any interventionist!) opened; consequently, it was decided to perform an interventional procedure without heparin.

Things do not always go as planned: the procedure was longer than expected and the patient developed what is dramatically illustrated in the next sequences. The patient sustained a thrombosis of the circumflex coronary artery extending to the left main stem that could not be effectively treated.

As we said earlier, in no circumstances should an intracoronary procedure (including an IVUS or Doppler or pressure wire evaluation) be performed without anticoagulating the patient.

> Even if the patient has a major allergy to heparin, action should be taken to institute appropriate antithrombin therapy. The slides that follow describe the types of heparin allergy that are clinically relevant and the appropriate anticoagulation therapy. The message is: for whatever reason never do an intervention without heparin. For the rare patient with heparin-induced thrombocytopenia use hirudine.

Massive air embolism

Case 22

This is really the worst-case scenario that can happen. I think very few people have seen or will see this type of complication because we always instinctively believe it will never happen. Unfortunately, these types of massive air embolism occur even in the best institutions. Be always on the alert: you need just one of this kind of complication to give you and your patient significant problems.

Instead of using dye, the ventriculogram was performed with 35ml of air. The patient immediately arrested and cardiopulmonary resuscitation (CPR) was continued for 45min without any improvement. Then came the bright idea to start percutaneous cardiopulmonary support (CPS). An external oxygenator with a centrifugal pump maintains full cardiac output and circulatory support. After 15min the patient regained cardiac function; after 2 days he awoke. The patient was discharged in good condition after 10 days.

> For massive air embolism consider CPS or any other form of extra corporeal circulation. Don't give up: these patients are still viable!

Carotid dissection with filter

Case 23

This case presents a complication caused by a filter device which was advanced into an internal carotid artery that was too tortuous for the flexibility of this particular filter device. The maneuver caused a dissection of the internal carotid artery, with flow limitation. It is important to distinguish between the complication as a true dissection and an image of a pseudo-dissection caused by spasm. The only way to make a definite diagnosis is to remove the filter. Sometimes, it may be important to advance a coronary wire, like a Balance 0.014" (Guidant, Temecula, CA), beyond the dissection before removing the filter. If we are dealing with a spasm, the removal of the filter will produce a clear amelioration of the flow, but not necessarily a prompt resolution. The local administration of nitroglycerin may be of help, but usually it is necessary to remove the filter device in order to reach a conclusion. In this case, no improvement was seen following the removal of the filter and a diagnosis of dissection was confirmed.

At this point, the faster approach needs to be instituted. Sealing the dissection with a coronary stent such as the Ultra (Guidant, Temecula, CA) 5mm diameter or the BX Velocity (Cordis, a Johnson and Johnson Company, Warren, NJ) 4mm diameter is the best solution.

Taking into account the rigidity of most current available carotid filters we suggest using the PercuSurge balloon on a wire device (Percusurge, Medtronic, Minneapolis, MN) when dealing with a tortuous carotid anatomy.

Complications during carotid surgery

The next two cases present what we can call "cath lab standby for carotid surgery".

Cases 24 and 25
These two cases show a massive intraoperative occlusive dissection with partial thrombosis that occurred very soon after the completion of a carotid endarterectomy in which the surgeon utilized the eversion technique. The procedure was initially performed without general anaesthesia. The surgeons became immediately aware of a developing neurological deficit. The patient was immediately transferred to the catheterization laboratory and a selective angiogram demonstrated thrombosis with possible dissection of the internal carotid artery. A Wallstent (Boston Scientific, Maple Grove, MN) was immediately positioned to reestablish a good lumen and flow.

The following case (Case 25) presents a similar problem but which was resolved with a different approach. This time, instead of performing a mechanical procedure to compress the thrombus and establish a good lumen, the operator elected to give a glycoprotein IIb/IIIa antagonist in order to resolve the thrombotic occlusion more satisfactorily. Unfortunately, the thrombus resolved but the intense antiplatelet activity of the above-mentioned approach, perhaps coupled with the sudden reperfusion of the brain, caused a massive intracerebral hemorrhage.

These two examples are included to show the potential benefit of an interventional procedure to correct a surgical complication, and to point out the unsettled treatment of carotid thrombosis with a potent antiplatelet or anticoagulant agent.

Disk 2
The value of IVUS

Introduction

Intravascular ultrasound (IVUS) is a device that is not essential in the catheterization laboratory. As a matter of fact, there are many cardiovascular centers performing a large number of coronary interventions with good results without any IVUS usage. Despite this fact, our view is that the possibility of investigating a lesion and evaluating the results of interventions with IVUS adds another parameter, thus making possible a more precise decision and enabling us to improve the result while maintaining safety.

One of the main concepts that are the basis for IVUS usage is achieving maximal stent expansion to avert stent thrombosis. In addition to a gain in short-term results, the largest possible lumen at the end of an intervention (with or without stenting) remains the most important and usable concept to lower the restenosis rate and, therefore, the need for further interventions on the treated lesion.

IVUS is particularly important in the following situations:

- treatment of long lesions in an attempt to minimize stent length, combining both optimal balloon angioplasty and optimal stenting, the so-called 'spot stenting;'
- treatment of lesions located on angiographic small vessels (<3 mm in diameter), when the index artery is supplying a large area of myocardium. The discordance between the small artery size and the large area of distribution may suggest that the vessel is a large one with diffuse disease. This initial impression needs to be confirmed by IVUS evaluation;
- further dilatation of a stent or a hard lesion when upsizing the balloon with high-pressure inflation becomes the next step to take in the procedure;
- treatment of in-stent restenosis, especially the diffuse type;
- evaluation of angiographically intermediate lesions or poorly defined lesions;

Of course, there are many other reasons and conditions in which IVUS may be useful and important; we have simply outlined the ones that direct most of our practice.

Unfortunately, IVUS is negatively affected by the added cost of the catheter and, more importantly, by the added time and device usage that an IVUS evaluation triggers. In addition, reading an IVUS examination, and making on-line evaluations and decisions, requires knowledge skills that can only be acquired with dedicated training.

In the brief section covered in this CD-ROM, we aim to give an overview of this field in order to stimulate more reading and to encourage in-field training and experience.

Case 26

This case illustrates the value of IVUS to determine the correct vessel size when the vessel is small when measured angiographically, while the anatomic distribution is large, thereby suggesting that the vessel is bigger.

Case 27

This case illustrates our concept of spot stenting to treat an area of long and diffuse disease. In the first slide, we see a diseased right coronary artery from the proximal part to the mid part of the vessel.

It is interesting to notice the discrepancy between the QCA vessel diameter, which is less than 3mm, and the media-to-media diameter measured with IVUS, which is over 4mm. The operator follows the IVUS measurements and uses a 3.75mm balloon. The reason for not using a 4mm balloon is mainly for safety: the operator does not fully match the IVUS diameter, especially when the discrepancy between the IVUS and angiographic measurements are large as in this case.

Following balloon dilatations, the IVUS catheter is inserted again. The goal is now to measure the cross-sectional area of the lumen in various segments. The segment with the luminal cross-sectional area that is less than 55% of the vessel cross-sectional area is considered an insufficient result, and it is therefore treated with stenting. Everything above that value is considered acceptable.

We also accept any absolute value of lumen cross-sectional area that is above 5.5mm^2.

The results shown in the third slide of this case show that in the proximal part of the artery, indicated by the arrow "A", the lumen cross-sectional area is only 3.5mm^2. The other segments are acceptable by the criteria just discussed.

For the above reason, a short stent is implanted in segment 'A,' while the other parts of the vessel are left alone.

The subsequent slides show the result after positioning the stent with an optimal lumen in 'A' and a persistent, acceptable lumen in the other segments of the vessels.

From this case, the conclusion is that we were able to treat a very long lesion with a relatively short stent implantation by combining angioplasty and stenting. This strategy is not only a strategy of IVUS-guided stenting, but also of IVUS-guided PTCA, with IVUS used as a decision-making tool.

Disk 3
Can I convince you that directional coronary atherectomy is still of value?

Introduction

Directional coronary atherectomy (DCA) prior to stenting is mainly performed to lower the risk of in-stent restenosis. This statement is quite radical and not yet supported by any large-scale randomized trial. The evidence so far comes from well-conducted registries and from data of two centers included in the AMIGO (Atherectomy before Multi-Link Improves Lumen Gain and Clinical Outcomes) Trial; the complete results of this large-scale randomized trial comparing DCA prior to stenting to stenting alone will be available in November 2001. Whatever the results of any trial that we are going to report, one fundamental assumption needs to be made clear: 'DCA does not work by the intention to treat.' This means that debulking up to a certain extent needs to be performed up to a certain extent in order to benefit from DCA. The amount of debulking we consider sufficient should be the one that leaves a <60% residual plaque area prior to stenting. An analysis of the SOLD (Stenting after Optimal Lesion Debulking) Registry found that when such optimal debulking was obtained, the loss index at follow-up after stenting, for lesions where an inferior amount of debulking was achieved, was only 0.28 compared to 0.52 (stenting without DCA) ($P=0.067$). The recent introduction of the new DCA device Flexicut (Guidant, Temecula, CA), which is compatible with an 8F guiding catheter, simplified some aspects of this procedure.

Despite this improvement, DCA remains an expensive, complex and more risky procedure compared to direct stenting. For all these reasons, DCA can only be recommended in situations where there is a clear, demonstrable cost-benefit in lowering restenosis. This cost should be calculated by taking into consideration the benefit of the procedure, such as the risk and the impact of having restenosis, versus the feasibility and complexity of the procedure itself. One example of benefit is the treatment of a stenosis located in:

- an unprotected non-calcified left main artery;
- an ostial or very proximal left anterior descending coronary artery;
- an ostial circumflex with a large area of distribution and 3.0–3.5mm in reference vessel size.

The need to lower restenosis in these specific situations is high and the complexity of performing DCA in a proximal lesion is acceptable. The insertion of an 8F balloon pump during the procedure adds a safety factor. A long lesion on a small posterolateral branch, an obtuse marginal branch, or in a medium-size right coronary artery has a high risk of restenosis. Still, the clinical impact of this event is not as dramatic or relevant as the prior example. Conversely, the performance of DCA in such a lesion is more complicated and not free of risk.

Most of the examples presented attempt to respect this rationale.

Case 28

This case illustrates a rather typical lesion, which in many centers could be well-treated with stenting, and most of the time with direct stenting. The angle of origin of the circumflex, which is at right-angles to the LAD, is in favor of an approach for stenting without any additional technique.

We performed directional atherectomy, followed by stenting, because our data suggest that the maximal lumen achieved with a combination of DCA and stenting gives the best assurance against restenosis. For this lesion located at the ostium of the left anterior descending, the risk of restenosis needs to be truly minimized.

Plaque shift toward the circumflex is usually less prominent if less plaque is available to be shifted.

Case 29

This is another typical example of a rather discrete lesion located at the ostium of the circumflex. Plaque debulking may lower the risk of plaque shift versus the LAD, in addition to lowering the risk of angiographic restenosis. For these reasons, this focal lesion was treated with atherectomy, followed by a very short stent implantation.

Case 30

This is a rather similar example of stenosis located at the ostium of the circumflex. Again, atherectomy is performed to minimize plaque shift and to provide a better lumen for stent implantation. The LAD is only mildly affected and undergoes low-pressure dilatation at the end of the procedure.

Case 31

This is a relatively unusual case. Here we have an image of restenosis (candy-wrapper type) that occurred a few months following radiation therapy. It is interesting to note that most of the radiated segments are perfectly normal but with this rather focal restenosis at the ostium of the LAD that also involves part of the left main stem. IVUS examinations confirm tissue proliferation rather than severe vessel remodeling as a cause of restenosis.

Case 32

This case shows extensive calcifications and diffuse disease of the left coronary system. The left main stem is severely narrowed up to the bifurcation of the circumflex and the LAD. The left anterior descending seems to be occluded in the third aspect of its length. The severe dilatation and the calcium present in the distal left main coronary artery demanded crossing of the lesion first with a balloon, then performing high-pressure dilatation, and finally a cutting balloon. Only following these steps were we able to advance an atherectomy device and remove a certain amount of tissue. It is interesting to see this device performing relatively well in challenging calcifications where directional atherectomy is usually not suited.

The final result is stabilized by placing a stent toward the LAD. The very favorable origin of the other branches did not demand a kissing inflation toward the circumflex and the intermediate branch.

Case 33

Here we have a nasty complication, which rarely occurs during or following directional atherectomy.

The operator should always be aware of this complication and the fact that problems can be solved if the regular true lumen is not lost. From this case, we understand the importance of obtaining a nice, complete image of the artery treated with direct atherectomy before removing the wire from the artery. The dissection extending from the ostium of the circumflex until the mid part of the vessel was treated by multiple stent implantations. From the IVUS medallion, it is interesting to see the haematoma and dissection lumen behind the stent struts.

Case 34

This is an illustration of an interesting approach that is frequently used in bifurcations, or even in trifurcations. The goal here is to stent most of the branches, leaving optimal access to all of them. For this reason, a stent is positioned right at the origin of the two branches. The technique that utilizes this approach is called 'skirt' or the pseudo-bifurcation technique.

In conclusion the following points concerning DCA need highlighting:

■ If you have any doubt concerning the patient's ability to tolerate the DCA procedure, based on the amount of myocardium at risk and on the baseline ejection fraction, do not hesitate to insert a balloon pump during the procedure. The balloon pump is removed at the end of the intervention and a sheath remains in the femoral artery. The patient will be able to return to his/her room;

■ Use a guiding catheter with a new, relaxed-type of curve for the left system; do not use a standard Judkins left coronary catheter.

■ Use guidewires with high support, such as the Ironman (Guidant, Temecula, CA) or the Platinum Plus (Boston Scientific, Boston, MA).

■ If the lesion is calcified following predilatation, the new Flexicut may still perform well with acceptable debulking.

Thrombus-containing lesions

Introduction

The presence of a thrombus detected by angiography cannot be dealt with by simple balloon angioplasty, or even direct stenting, because the thrombus will break into small fragments or, thanks to the stent struts, plaster the material to the vessel wall. The risk and the consequences of distal embolizations are present and will impact on the prognosis of the patient. The modern operator needs to be aware of this and act in a specific manner when confronted with these types of lesions.

The conjunctive use of pharmacologic and mechanical protection is frequently necessary. Pretreatment with Gp IIb/IIIa antagonists needs to be complemented with the use of a mechanical device specifically made to deal with thrombotic lesions.

These devices can be divided into two categories:

■ thrombus removal devices such as Angiojet (Possis Medical, Minneapolis, MN), X-Sizer (Endicor Medical, Valkenswaard, The Netherlands) or the Rescue (Boston Scientific, Maple Grove, MN),

■ protection devices such as filters or an occlusive balloon on a wire with thrombus removal possibility (PercuSurge, Medtronic, Indianapolis MN).

In which situations the operator needs to use one device versus the other depends on personal experience, the amount of thrombus present, and device availability. We cannot exclude that some circumstances may demand the use of two devices, such as a thrombus removal device and a protection device.

> The bottom line: a thrombotic lesion requires specific treatment that is aimed at protecting the distal vascular bed and supplying the myocardium.

Cases 35–37 are all aimed to demonstrate this area of use.

Case 35

This is a very nice iconographic example of how large vessels are prone to blood clotting.

The clinical circumstances tell us that most of the occlusion of the right coronary artery may be thrombotic. The operator correctly decided to use a thrombus suction device. The device was advanced up to the distal right coronary artery and then was activated. Following a few passes, a distal flow was obtained that was sufficient to see the distal peripheral vessel anatomy and perform multiple stenting.

Case 36

This is an unusual case of a thrombus-containing lesion. The lesion deviates from the usual clinical context in which we are used to seeing a thrombotic lesion. As a matter of fact this is not a true thrombotic lesion: rather, it is an embolic occlusion.

The patient came to the hospital following sudden onset of chest pain and ST elevation in II, III, aVF and V4–6. Following the initial angiogram, it was clear that there was a distal occlusion of the left anterior descending which did not resolve following passage of the guidewire. The history of an intermittent atrial fibrillation history made the operator suppose that an embolic myocardial infarction was the primary cause for this occlusion. A thrombus-removing device, the Rescue catheter (Boston Scientific, Maple Grove, MN), was effectively used in this specific patient.

Case 37

This is an example of an acute myocardial infarction, cause by a thrombotic occlusion on the distal circumflex. Ballooning of this occlusion or subocclusion was followed by slow flow. Nitroprusside partially improved this event, but the reestablishment of a distal flow was obtained subsequent only to repeated inflations up to the very proximal circumflex.

Coronary ruptures

Introduction

> It is very difficult to perform complex coronary interventions and to strive for optimal stenting without having experienced a coronary rupture.

Operators who have not encountered a rupture obviously should continue not to do so. I also think that if you have had a coronary rupture in your experience, as long as this complication stays at very low levels (<1% with contemporary tools), you should not necessarily feel you are at discordance with optimal technique.

The table presented here divides ruptures according to their extent.

Rupture after DCA and following rotablation with subsequent positioning of a covered stent

Cases 38 and 39
These two cases fit into the category of major ruptures, with contrast media moving outside from the coronary wall.

A number of ruptures we are showing have a common denominator: the use of a compliant or semicompliant balloon, inflated at high pressure in a rigid or calcified lesion. This action may lead to vessel rupture at the lesion site or at the margins of the lesion. When a compliant balloon is constrained at a site of incomplete expansion, high-pressure inflation will over-expand the unconstrained segments of the balloon to an extent larger than the defined pressure–volume relation for the specific balloon. Any case of coronary rupture will become a real major complication, with further difficulties arising if the patient has been treated with GPIIb/IIIa inhibitors. This fact needs to be foremost in the operator's mind when inflating a balloon at high pressure for a stent positioned in a lesion that is difficult to dilate. The other important element to consider is the importance of paying close attention to the IVUS measurements.

> In any situation in which the operator is treating a very hard lesion, one that does not expand at high pressure, an IVUS examination should be performed before moving to a bigger balloon.

Another practical message is: in case of major ruptures (type 3 ruptures) the threshold to use a polytetrafluoroethylene (PTFE)-covered stent (JOMED, Rangendingen, Germany) should be low. In these situations, the possibility of sealing the large opening in the vessel wall with prolonged balloon inflation is dependent on full reversal of heparin with protamine, and on the possibility of performing a prolonged balloon inflation. Unfortunately, these two actions do not interact well with each other. With the availability of a premounted PTFE stent, it is possible to seal the rupture even without fully reversing the heparin.

In one of the cases presented, a PTFE-covered stent was deployed too late in the course of events. The full reversal of heparin and the prolonged ischemia caused by the continuous balloon inflation, with slow flow into the distal bed, contributed to the early thrombosis of the covered stent.

Distal guidewire perforation

Case 40
This case shows a distal guidewire perforation that occurred while obtaining the last final angiograms at the end of the procedure. The guidewire was intentionally advanced distally in order to partially remove the big guiding catheter from the ostium of the left main stem. This maneuver is frequently performed in the practice of interventional cardiology. To make the problem more difficult to solve, the patient was pretreated with abciximab.

For these types of distal perforations, the solutions available are:

- very distal embolization utilizing coils or thrombogenic material injected from a dedicated catheter positioned distally, or even from the lumen of a coaxial balloon;
- exclusion of the branch from which the bleeding originates by placing a covered stent, thus sealing the branch.

Sealing of a leaking side branch by excluding the branch with a PTFE-covered stent

Case 41
The second possible solution for the distal perforation presented in the previous case is well demonstrated in this rupture, which originates from the distal end of a branch of the right coronary artery. The operator decided to place a PTFE-covered stent (JOMED, Rangendingen, Germany) to exclude the branch feeding the perforation completely.

Rupture of a vein graft

Case 42
Rupture of a vein graft can be managed with a covered stent unless there is complete or severe separation of the extremities of the ruptured segment. In this last and most dramatic condition, the only approach is to seal the proximal stump of the vein graft completely with coils.

Disk 4

1 Overview of cutting balloon angioplasty: general presentation

2 Cutting balloon angioplasty: areas of application

Introduction

The cutting balloon is a device that has been resurrected. In-stent restenosis is its major application, and the lack of 'watermelon seeding effect' is the most immediate reward following use of the cutting balloon.

> Compared to the traditional teaching regarding cutting balloon angioplasty, the new usage of this device introduced the concept of high-pressure inflations (up to 12atm) and of multiple inflations.

Following treatment of in-stent restenosis with the cutting balloon, there are some registries and single center experiences reporting a lower incidence of new restenosis. Randomized trials are being carried out in this area and more definitive data will soon be available.

> In addition to treating in-stent restenosis, the cutting balloon appears of interest in the treatment of:
>
> - lesions located in small vessels;
> - fibrocalcific lesions;
> - ostial lesions;
> - some bifurcational lesions.

Cases 43–47 illustrate the aforementioned lesions. At the present time, the application of the cutting balloon to these areas is supported by the experience of different operators, and by registries or case reports. Unfortunately, it will be difficult to design specific studies addressing those areas of application.

Case 43

Illustrated here is a rather unique application of the cutting balloon. Following stent implantation in the proximal LAD, the stent could not be fully expanded in its distal part, even at 30atm. An attempt to advance a cutting balloon was made, with single inflation at 12atm without an immediate improvement in the result. The high-pressure balloon was placed again and fully expanded at 28atm.

Regular angioplasty was performed on the mid left anterior descending and on the circumflex.

Case 44

This case illustrates an unusual application of the cutting balloon that is used for stent post-dilatation. It is not clear how the cutting balloon might achieve what a high-pressure balloon is unable to do. It is possible that the more even force distribution of the cutting balloon (due to the presence of the metallic blades) may create plaque ruptures in an area where a standard balloon does not exert the same force.

It is interesting to look at the IVUS images in the left anterior descending following the use of different-sized cutting balloons and various pressures that cause a significant gain in the lumen cross-sectional area.

The baseline IVUS evaluation shows a severe calcification with 360° calcium in two cross-sections. An initial dilatation with a conservative strategy utilizing a 3mm cutting balloon is performed in various segments of the left anterior descending. Subsequently, the mid part of the vessel is treated with the Carbostent (Sorin Biomedica SPA, Saluggia, Italy)(2.5mm diameter, 25mm long). The decision was taken because the result following angioplasty and evaluation IVUS was unsatisfactory.

Owing to the presence of severe calcification with diffuse disease and taking advantage of the large size of the proximal vessel, another Carbostent (3.5mm diameter, 15mm long) is implanted proximally. Following implantation of the two stents, IVUS imaging showed an insufficient result in the most distal part of the vessel. Another stent, 3mm in diameter, is implanted at this level. Lesions in the mid LAD and in the diagonal branch are then treated with regular angioplasty. A final IVUS evaluation showed a persistent and insufficient result in the proximal and distal part of the vessel.

Now comes the novelty. A cutting balloon, 3.5mm in diameter, was inflated at high pressure in the proximal segment; this was followed by a larger cutting balloon (4mm) inflated at the ostium of the LAD. It is interesting that this second balloon is inflated inside the recently deployed stent. The lumen cross-sectional area in this stent increased from $5.4mm^2$ to $7.5mm^2$. A similar phenomenon occurs in the very distal part of the vessel.

Following a dilatation with the Solaris balloon at high pressure, the stent lumen cross-sectional area is still below $3mm^2$. Only the use of a cutting balloon 3mm in diameter inflated at 14atm was able to increase the lumen cross-sectional area to over $4mm^2$.

Case 45

As a tribute to the synergy of different devices, we present this case of a young lady with diabetes mellitus and diffuse disease in the major coronary arteries.

In particular, the left anterior descending is totally occluded in the mid part. IVUS evaluation confirms that we are not dealing with a very small vessel, as the angiography suggests. The vessel is over 3.5mm in diameter.

At this point, most of the proximal part of the vessel is dilated with multiple inflations utilizing a 3.5mm cutting balloon. The procedure is completed with implantation of a 3.5mm diameter, 17mm long Quanam-paclitaxel derivate sleeve coated stent (Quanam Medical Corporation, Santa Clara, CA).

The decision to implant this type of stent is due to a very high risk of restenosis in a diabetic patient with a diffusely diseased angiographically small vessel that was totally occluded.

In order to maximize the result, another stent was implanted in the very proximal part of the LAD. It is interesting to notice that a small gap was left between the two stents.

At 6-month follow-up the site of this small gap underwent negative remodeling and proliferation. Moreover, it is also interesting to observe the complete absence of hyperplasia inside the two drug-coated stents.

The patient was subsequently treated with a short stent implantation to cover the gap between the two stents.

Case 46

This case shows the combination of two strategies to treat a lesion con-sidered at high risk for restenosis. This lesion is located at the ostium of the LAD. The vessel is first optimally predilated with a cutting balloon and then a so-called 'smart stent' is implanted at the ostium of the LAD. This is a drug-coated stent utilizing a sleeve with paclitaxel derivate on it. As shown in other sections of *Tips and Tricks*, this type of lesion could have been treated with directional atherectomy and stenting.

The readers should note the severe narrowing present at the ostium of the circumflex following stenting of the LAD. This severe narrowing required implantation of a regular stent (the study protocol did not allow implantation of two drug-coated stents in two different vessels). The final result is more than acceptable, but with potential for restenosis in the metal stent. In addition, the IVUS images show that the true ostium of the circumflex is not fully covered by the stent.

The follow-up at 6 months shows a not unexpected restenosis at the ostium of the circumflex and a surprising new lesion at the distal edge of the drug-coated stent. It is our impression that possible trauma of the long deploying balloon contributed to this distal stenosis. The operator implanted a short stent to solve this problem.

The ostium of the circumflex was treated with simple angioplasty. It is not completely clear why the operator chose this option rather than the cutting balloon. A possible interpretation is related to the risk of the cutting balloon being trapped in some struts of the stent present in the left anterior descending.

This safe approach is frequently advocated, especially with a stent positioned in the left main coronary artery or in the proximal LAD.

Case 47

This case illustrates a rather unusual phenomenon: the occurrence of slow flow following re-PTCA for in-stent restenosis. The important aspect of this case is the prompt and rather dramatic improvement following selective injection of nitroprusside.

In our experience the occurrence of slow flow in cases of in-stent restenosis is rare. Treatment of this complication with direct and selective injections of nitroprusside is still the most effective approach.

Appendix

Stent selection

Antonio Colombo and Goran Stankovic

Ever since the data from the Belgian–Netherlands Stent (BENESTENT) study[1] and the Stent Restenosis Study (STRESS)[2] became available, and with the elimination of anticoagulant therapy after stent implantation,[3–5] the implantation of coronary stents became an integral part of most interventional procedures of percutaneous revascularization.

The growth in stent implantation stimulated the commercial introduction of a number of different stents. Table I illustrates the characteristics of most of the stents available in the year 2001. The rapid increase in the number of designs available is such that any list rapidly becomes outdated. Table I shows that some stent designs are quite similar to others, although with some diversities. The reasons why different designs have been proposed are multiple. Besides the need to overcome a specific patent, there are conceptual grounds that have stimulated inventors to introduce new designs. The need to increase the flexibility to allow better and safer stent delivery is one of the most important reasons for improving a stent design. Manufacturers try to achieve this goal without compromising either radial support or lesion coverage. Another element, not specifically part of the design yet still very specific to the stent, is its radiological visibility.

Many of these design characteristics were not introduced with the idea of making a stent more suitable for a specific lesion. Every stent manufacturer is likely to assume that its stent will be employed for the largest possible number of lesions.

This chapter focuses on the specific features of stent design: what makes a specific stent more suitable or less suitable for a particular type of lesion or anatomy?

Types of stent

Stents can be classified according to their mechanism of expansion (self-expanding, balloon expandable), their composition (stainless steel, cobalt-based alloy, tantalum, nitinol, inert coating, active coating,

Table 1 *Stent engineering data.*

Brand	Manufacturer	Structure	Material	Strut (wire) thickness (mm)	Metal/artery (%)*
AVE S670	Medtronic	sinusoidal ring	stainless steel	0.127	19
AVE S7	Medtronic	sinusoidal ring	stainless steel	0.102	17–23
BeStent 2	Medtronic	slotted tube	stainless steel	0.085–0.095	12–17
BiodivYsio AS	Biocompatibles	slotted tube	stainless steel	0.091	19–25
BiodivYsio OC	Biocompatibles	slotted tube	stainless steel	0.091	9–12
BX Velocity	Cordis J&J	slotted tube	stainless steel	0.14	15
BX Sonic	Cordis J&J	slotted tube	stainless steel	0.14	15
Carbostent Sirius	Sorin	slotted tube	stainless steel	0.075	12–17
Cook V-Flex	Cook	slotted tube	stainless steel	0.07	15
Diamond Flex AS	Phytis	slotted tube	stainless steel	0.075	10–18
JOSTENT Flex	JOMED	slotted tube	stainless steel	0.09	16
JOSTENT Plus	JOMED	slotted tube	stainless steel	0.09	16
JOSTENT Graft	JOMED	slotted tube	stainless steel	0.20	100
LP Stent	Boston Scientific	slotted tube	stainless steel	0.1	15
Mac Carbon Stent	AMG	slotted tube	stainless steel	0.085	8–15
Multi-Link Tetra	Guidant	slotted tube	stainless steel	0.091–0.124	12–20
Multi-Link Penta	Guidant	slotted tube	stainless steel	0.091–0.124	12–16
Multi-Link Ultra	Guidant	slotted tube	stainless steel	0.127	15–25
NIR 7-cells & 9-cells	Medinol, Boston Scientific	multicell design	stainless steel	0.1	11–18
NIR Royal	Medinol, Boston Scientific	multicell design	stainless steel, gold	0.1	11–18
P-S 153	Cordis J&J	slotted tube	stainless steel	0.062	18
PURA A	Devon	slotted tube	stainless steel	0.12	10–15
PURA Vario AL	Devon	slotted tube	stainless steel	0.07	10–18
PURA Vario AS	Devon	slotted tube	stainless steel	0.07	10–18
Teneo Tenax-XR	Biotronik	slotted tube	stainless steel	0.08	14–22
Tsunami	Terumo	slotted tube	stainless steel	0.08	18
Small vessel stents					
AVE S660	Medtronic AVE	sinusoidal ring	stainless steel	0.127	20
BeStent (4-crowns)	Medtronic AVE	slotted tube	stainless steel	0.085–0.095	12–17
BiodivYsio SV	Biocompatibles	slotted tube	stainless steel	0.05	9
BX Velocity	Cordis J&J	slotted tube	stainless steel	0.14	15
Carbostent Sirius 4-cell	Sorin	slotted tube	stainless steel	0.075	12–17
JOSTENT Flex	JOMED	slotted tube	stainless steel	0.09	16
JOSTENT Plus	JOMED	slotted tube	stainless steel	0.09	16
Multi-Link Pixel	Guidant ACS	slotted tube	stainless steel	0.099	15
PURA Vario AS	Devon	slotted tube	stainless steel	0.07	10–18

*Does not necessarily mean vessel wall coverage.

biodegradable), and their design (mesh structure, coil, slotted tube, ring, multidesign, custom design; see Table 1). According to the manufacturers, all stents are suitable for implantation in native coronary arteries of appropriate size, and the indications for the Palmaz–Schatz stent have recently been expanded to lesions located in vein grafts. No stent is specifically designed for implantation in a particular lesion, and the absolute or relative contraindications to the use of stents apply to

Recoil (%)	Foreshortening (%)	Radioopacity	Markers	Lengths (mm)	Diameters (mm)
3	3	medium	no	9, 12, 15, 18, 24, 30	3.0, 3.5, 4.0
2	3	medium	no	9, 12, 15, 18, 24, 30	3.0, 3.5, 4.0
2	0	low	yes	9, 12, 15, 18, 24, 30	2.5, 3.0, 3.5, 4.0
2	4	low	no	11, 15	3.0, 3.5, 4.0
4	4	low	no	15, 18, 22, 28	3.0, 3.5, 4.0
2.5	2	medium	no	8, 13, 18, 23, 28, 32	2.25, 2.5, 2.75, 3.0, 3.5, 4.0
2.4	1.7	medium	no	8, 13, 18, 23, 28, 33	2.25, 2.5, 2.75, 3.0, 3.5, 4.0
3–5	0	low	yes	9, 12, 15, 19, 25	2.5, 3.0, 3.5, 4.0
21	0	low	no	12, 16, 20, 24	2.5, 3.0, 3.5
3–5	1	low	no	9, 12, 16, 20, 25	2.5, 3.0, 3.5, 4.0
4	5	low	no	9, 16, 26, 32	2.0, 2.5, 3.0, 3.5, 4.0, 4.5
4	5	low	no	9, 17, 27, 33	2.0, 2.5, 3.0, 3.5, 4.0, 4.5
2	3	high	no	9, 12, 16, 19, 26	2.5, 3.0, 3.5, 4.0, 4.5, 5.0
2	3–5	low	no	8, 12, 18, 24	2.5, 30, 3.5, 4.0
3	1	low	no	9, 13, 17, 22	2.0, 2.5, 3.0, 3.5, 4.0, 4.5
2–3	3–4	medium	no	8, 13, 18, 23, 28	2.5, 2.75, 3.0, 3.5, 4.0
2–3	3–4	medium	no	8, 13, 15, 18, 23, 28, 33	2.75, 3.0, 3.5, 4.0
2	5	medium	no	13, 18, 28, 38	3.5, 4.0, 4.5, 5.0
3	3	low	no	9, 16, 25, 32	2.0, 2.5, 3.0, 3.5, 4.0, 4.5, 5.0
5	3	high	no	9, 16, 25, 32	2.0, 2.5, 3.0, 3.5, 4.0, 4.5, 5.0
5	8	medium	no	8, 9, 14, 18	3.0, 3.5, 4.0
2	1–5	low	no	7, 15	3.0, 3.5, 4.0, 4.5, 5.0
3	5	low	no	6, 10, 16, 24, 28	3.5, 4.0
3	7	low	no	6, 10, 16, 24, 28	2.5, 3.0
5	3	low	yes	10, 15, 20, 25, 30	2.5, 3.0, 3.5, 4.0
5	5	low	no	10, 15, 20, 30	2.5, 3.0, 3.5, 4.0
2	1.5	medium	no	9, 12, 15, 18, 24	2.5
1.6–2.2	0	low	yes	9, 12, 15, 18, 24, 30	2.5
1	4	low	no	10, 15, 18	2.0, 2.5
2.5	2	low	no	8, 13, 18, 23, 28, 32	2.25, 2.5, 2.75
3–5	0	low	yes	9, 12, 15, 19, 25	2.5
4	5	low	no	9, 16, 26, 32	2.0, 2.5
4	5	low	no	9, 17, 27, 33	2.0, 2.5
4	11	medium	no	8, 13, 18, 23, 28	2.25, 2.5
3	7	low	no	6, 10, 16, 24, 28	2.5

stents in general and not to a specific stent. Possible exceptions are the Multi-Link Ultra stent (Guidant, Temecula, CA), which is more specifically designed for vein graft implantation with a 9-cell design versus the 6-cell design of the Multi-Link Tetra. The JOMED polytetrafluoroethylene (PTFE)-covered stent (JOMED, Rangendingen, Germany) is specifically made for certain types of application (coronary ruptures, aneurysms, saphenous vein grafts).

Table 2 *Crossing profile*

Brand	Manufacturer	Crossing profile (mm)*	
		2.5mm diameter	3.0mm diameter
AVE S670	Medtronic		1.09
AVE S660	Medtronic	0.99	
BeStent 2	Medtronic	1.07	1.17
BiodivYsio AS	Biocompatibles		1.07
BiodivYsio SV	Biocompatibles	0.84	
BX Velocity	Cordis J&J	1.07	1.17
BX Sonic	Cordis J&J	1.09	1.14
Carbostent	Sorin	1.02	1.04
Multi-Link Tetra	Guidant ACS	1.04	1.12
Multi-Link Penta	Guidant ACS		1.07
NIR with socks	Medinol, Boston Scientific	1.09	1.12
Multi-Link Pixel	Guidant ACS	0.93	

*These data reflect measurements performed by individual manufacturers; the methodology used to measure and the exact site of measurements may differ among different stents.

Different characteristics, such as strut thickness, metal to artery ratio, degree of radio-opacity, degree of foreshortening and recoil of a number of currently used stents are shown in Table 1. All stents now are available premounted on dedicated delivery systems.

> The capacity of a stent to cross a lesion does not depend solely on a crossing profile (Table 2) but also on:
>
> - the amount of friction of the stent itself,
> - flaring of the distal struts upon friction with the lesion,
> - flexibility of the stent and of the delivery balloon,
> - pushability of the delivery system.
>
> For all these reasons, it is not surprising that a stent with a larger crossing profile may cross a lesion more easily than a stent with a smaller crossing profile.

We now describe the selective use of different stents in different lesions.

Most coronary lesions

In the past we categorized a specific stent for proximal and not angulated lesions, while other stents were mainly reserved for tortuous anatomies and complex situations. There are no doubts that some stents are more flexible than others – with a smaller profile and therefore more deliverable. Still, these extra features become necessary only in very selected situations. Consequently, with some exceptions, most stents currently available are suitable almost for any type of coronary lesion. We will discuss the exceptions separately. The stents to be used in 'most coronary lesions' are the new slotted tubular stents and some new designs of ring stent. The lesion coverage, the recoil, and the risk of plaque prolapse are reduced with this type of design. These features are important for offering the largest possible final diameter. Currently, the achievement of a large final lumen diameter remains the most solid approach to limiting restenosis.[6]

The Palmaz–Schatz stent led the way, and gave the baton to the BX Velocity (Cordis, a J&J Company, Warren, NJ; the Venus Trial: a multi-center registry of the Cordis BX Velocity stent),[7] and we should not be surprised if very soon the BX Velocity were to be replaced by the sirolimus-coated BX Velocity.[8] The BX Velocity can be considered the stent for everyday usage, with only a few conditions in which it may not be ideal. The BX Velocity is available with three different patterns of cells, according to the vessel size in which the stent will be implanted: 6 cells for vessels up to 3mm, 7 cells for vessels up to 4mm; and 9 cells for vessels up to 5mm.

Similar considerations apply to the Multi-Link Tetra (Guidant, Temecula, CA). The overall performance of these two stents is similar, with only selected situations where one of them (probably the Tetra) is more deliverable. The unique feature of the Tetra delivery system (similar for the Ultra) is its shaft length of 143cm which is 3cm longer than the BX Velocity, while all the other delivery systems are 138 or 135cm long.

The careful observer may find more stent-to-vessel conformability with the Tetra stent, but nobody knows if this feature bears any clinical implication. Preserving the original shear stress at various levels of the arterial segment may lower the amount of tissue hyperplasia.[9]

The NIR stent (Medinol, Jerusalem, Israel and Scimed, Boston Scientific, Maple Grove, MN), with its new socks delivery system, is another important stent to be considered for the everyday lesion. The excellent plaque coverage given by the design of this stent is an advantage to consider in lesions prone to plaque prolapse. This factor should be kept in mind when dealing with a vessel with a reference diameter ≥4mm. As the NIR stent is available with 7 cells and 9 cells (Figure 1) structure is an important attribute for its usage in large vessels, including saphenous vein grafts. The socks delivery system protects the stent while it is being negotiated through calcium and while crossing another stent. These features are unique to this type of stent and, even better, to this type of delivery system.

The performance of this stent was evaluated against the Palmaz–Schatz stent in the NIRVANA (NIR Vascular Advanced North American trial) randomized study.[10] This trial reported a follow-up restenosis rate of 19.3% for the NIR stent and 22.4% for the Palmaz–Schatz stent. The

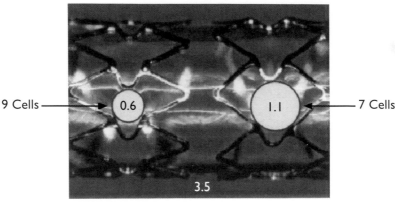

9 Cells ——→ 0.6   1.1 ←—— 7 Cells

3.5

Cell Diameter of 3mm Expanded Stent

Figure 1 *The NIR stent (Medinol, Jerusalem, Israel, and Boston Scientific, Maple Grove, MN). Comparison of 7- and 9-cell designs.*

moderate rigidity of the NIR stent discourages its implantation through very tortuous segments and on lesions located at severe bends, because this stent may give a hinge effect, which has been associated with an increase in restenosis.[11] Figure 2 demonstrate this hinge effect caused by an NIR stent, which becomes rigid upon deployment. This particular lesion restenosed 4 months later at the distal extremity of the stent (Figure 3). The operator should be aware of these situations and select a different type of stent.

The good features of these three stents are related to the delivery balloon:

- the perfect retention, which has almost eliminated the problem of stent loss;
- the minimal hangover of the delivery balloon from the stent, which limits the trauma and the risk of peristent dissections;
- the low compliance, which assures a more homogeneous stent deployment (Figure 4).

The BeStent (Medtronic AVE, Minneapolis, MN), and now the BeStent 2 with a closer strut design, is another stent to consider. The unique feature of this stent, the presence of proximal and distal gold markers, allows very precise placement. Another feature of the BeStent (not the BeStent 2) is the presence of a large or open cell design that facilitates the access to side branches.

The BiodivYsio stent (Biocompatibles, Galway, Ireland) is another good stent with optimal scaffolding to be considered for most lesions. This stent is available also with an open cell design that is suitable for lesions involving the origin of side braches. Compared with the open cell design, the added support design has an extra strut between interlock-

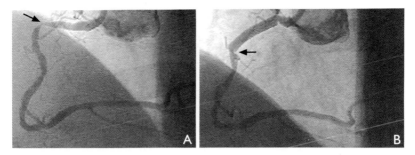

Figure 2 *A, Baseline angiogram of a lesion (arrow) in the proximal right coronary artery; B, After implantation of a 9-cell, 16mm long NIR stent. The hinge site at the end of the stent is clear (arrow).*

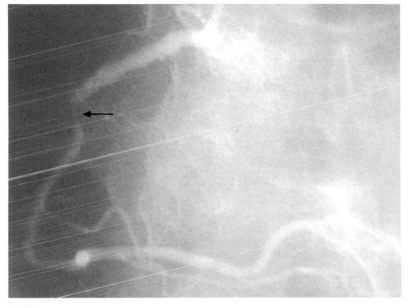

Figure 3 *Follow-up angiogram of the lesion in Figure 2 4 months later, showing restenosis at the hinge site (arrow).*

ing arrowheads which provides greater paving function for lesions where additional support is required (Figure 5).

The BiodivYsio stent was recently evaluated against the Duet stent (Guidant, Temecula, CA) in a randomized trial (DISTINCT: BiodivYsio Stent IN randomized Control Trial). Both stents showed an excellent low restenosis rate of 19% in selected favorable lesions. It is our impression that the standard BiodivYsio stent delivery system is more rigid than other stents and not so ideal for tortuous anatomies. New versions of the delivery system will soon be released to overcome this potential limitation. The availability of a small vessels design of this stent, which is very trackable and with a low profile, should be kept in mind when confronted with complex anatomy.

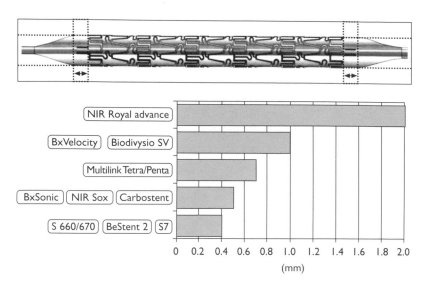

Figure 4 *Length of balloon protrusion for common-usage stents (mm).*

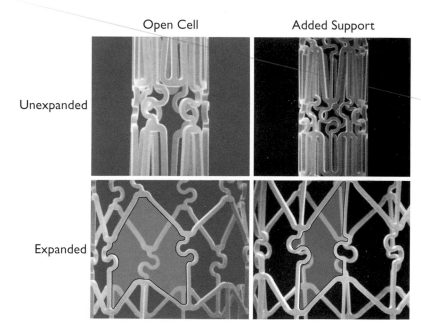

Figure 5 *The BiodivYsio stent (Biocompatibles, Galway, Ireland). Comparison of open cell and added support designs.*

A unique feature of the BiodivYsio family is their phosphorylcholine coating that lowers platelet adhesion to the stent struts and may be used as a platform for drug delivery.

Among the ring stents the new S7 (Medtronic AVE, Minneapolis, MN) appears an improvement compared with the S670, with more plaque coverage and an angiographic appearance very similar to the slotted tubular stents. This stent can be considered good for most lesions. In addition, the flexibility, conformability, and lower friction typical of the ring design of the S7 gives this stent an added bonus for deliverability in complex anatomies or through a stent.

Among the stainless steel stents with a good track record, we cannot dismiss the family of the PURA (Devon Medical, Hamburg, Germany) and the V-Flex plus (Cook, Broomfield, CO). We tested these stents in our laboratory and confirmed a good mechanical performance with a clinical outcome very similar to well-known stents.

To make the choice more difficult the interventionist is confronted with some other excellent stents such as the Sorin Sirius Carbostent (Sorin Biomedica Cardio, Saluggia, Italy). This stent performs quite well in different anatomies and lesions, has platinum end markers, and is covered with a thin layer of turbostatic carbon to lower interaction with platelets. A recent report from a registry, showing a restenosis rate of 11% and a bimodal distribution of the loss index,[12] raises the possibility of enhanced biocompatibility for subjects with an allergy to metal contaminants present in stainless steel.[13] At least four other carbon-coated stents are currently available in Europe: the BioDiamond (Plasma Chem, Mainz, Germany), the Diamond Flex (Phytis, Dreieich, Germany), the MAC Carbon Stent (AMG, Raesfeld-Erle, Germany), and the Tenax (Biotronik, Berlin, Germany). Dedicated randomized trials are in progress to test advantages that these inert coated stents may have over the stainless steel stents.

Lesions situated on a curve (≥90°) or immediately followed by a curve

No specific study has examined this issue.

> In view of the straightening effect caused by a slotted tubular stent and the possible consequences on restenosis, the operator should consider using a stent that conforms better to the original anatomy.

While no formal contraindication for any type of stent can be made, our preference is for stents that tend to better conform to the anatomy of the vessels. The traditional ring design, such as the S670, is quite conformable but it may allow too much plaque protrusion when opened in a curved segment; the new S7 is a clear improvement. Thin-strut slotted tubular stents are also quite conformable (PURA AS and AL 0.07,

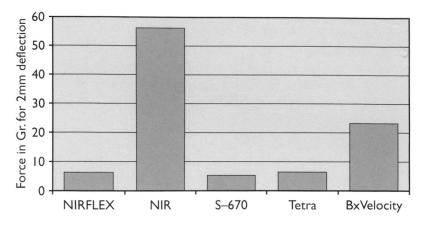

Figure 6 *Stent conformability. (Courtesy of Kobi Richter, Medinol, Jerusalem, Israel).*

BeStent 0.075mm, Sorin Carbostent 0.075mm, Tenax 0.08mm, BiodivYsio 0.09mm, Jostent 0.09mm). Strut thickness is not the only variable that may affect conformability: the specific stent design may be more important. For example, the NIR stent, which is thinner (0.1mm) than the BX Velocity (0.14mm) has a lower conformability (Figure 6). The Multi-Link Tetra is a variable-thickness stent (0.091–0.124mm), with excellent conformability.

Recently we had the opportunity to evaluate the new version of the NIR stent: NIRflex. We have been impressed by the excellent conformability without plaque protrusion demonstrated by this new stent design (Figure 7).

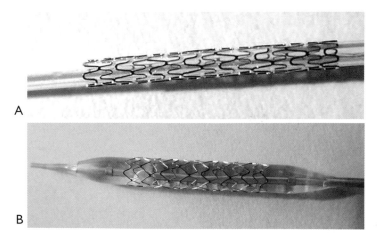

Figure 7 *The NIR Flex stent (Medinol, Jerusalem, Israel, and Boston Scientific, Maple Grove, MN). A, Mounted on balloon; B, expanded with the 3mm balloon at 10atm.*

Ostial lesions

Ostial lesions are classified as either aorto-ostial or coronary–ostial.

> For aorto-ostial lesions, the slotted tubular design, preferably with strong radial support and radiologic visibility, is the most appropriate one.[14]

New ring designs, such as the S670 and S7, are also appropriate.

The recent availability of stents with end markers may improve the precise positioning. As these stents belong to the thin strut group of stents, we prefer their implantation at the coronary–ostial rather than the aorto-ostial location. The presence of the aorta with a lot of elastic recoil in our view favors the usage of a stronger and thicker strut type of stent when dealing with lesions involving the true coronary ostia or the aortic insertion of a saphenous vein graft.

Unfortunately, even with optimal lesions, predilatation, and associated debulking, the restenosis rate in the aorto-ostial lesions continues to be a problem.[15,16]

It is interesting to consider the usage of the JOMED PTFE-covered stent (JOMED, Rangendingen, Germany) for the aorto-ostial location. No data are available in the literature, and our preliminary experience has not been very encouraging.

Regarding the implantation of the NIR Royal in these types of lesions, we maintain a conservative attitude as we await the results of the recently performed randomized trial of the NIR Royal versus the NIR Primo stent (NIR Ultimate Gold-Gilded Equivalency Trial: NUGGET). This consideration comes after a recent publication showed a high restenosis rate with the gold-coated In-flow stent.[17]

For aorto-ostial lesions with a reference vessel size 4mm in diameter or larger, we prefer: the BX Velocity, the 9-cell NIR, the Ultra, or the JOMED PTFE-covered stent.

Bifurcational lesions

The most important element in stent implantation in a bifurcational lesion is to decide whether (1) both branches of the bifurcation need to receive stents or (2) only the major one needs a stent while the other branch is dilated through the deployed stent.

The goal is to try not to implant stents in both branches. Implanting two stents adds cost, complexity, and possible complications to the procedure without any advantage in terms of angiographic restenosis or long-term events.[18]

The real issue is that this procedure does not improve the long-term
outcome of the patient. Placement of the stent in the large branch and
dilating into the small one remains the most practical solution. When this
approach is not appropriate, or a flow or lumen compromising dissection occurs in the side branch, both branches require stent implantation.

If we start the approach with the goal of stenting only the main branch,
we prefer a stent with large side openings among the cells and, even
more important, with cells that can be well opened following the
passage of a balloon into the side branch. Figure 8 shows some slotted
tube stents with the cross-sectional area of the cell following stent
dilatation and with the cross-sectional area of the same cell following
maximal opening with a balloon inflated into the side branch.

The rather closed cell design of the NIR does not allow significant expansion of the opening toward the side branch even after crossing and inflating a balloon. If, for whatever reason, the operator decides to use an NIR
stent the 7-cell stent should be used instead of the 9-cell (Figure 1).

As we mentioned earlier, there is the option of using a stent with a
large side opening, such as the BiodivYsio open cell design (Figure 5) or
the S670. The advantage of this decision is that the initial access to the
side branch is facilitated. A possible disadvantage is incomplete prolapse
of one strut toward the side branch following the kissing balloon dilatation. The concept of strut prolapse from the main branch toward the
side branch has been pioneered by Dr Marie Claude Morice and Dr
Tierry Lefevre and named 'stenting both branches with one stent.'
When the design is very open there is less possibility for a strut to
straddle toward the side branch. Slotted tubular stents that maximally
demonstrated this feature are the BeStent and the Carbostent; the BX
Velocity and the Tetra are also quite adequate (Figure 9). Whatever
stent the operator uses it is important to perform a kissing balloon
inflation at the end of the procedure to correct for the stent distortion
that occurs following the balloon inflation in the side branch.[19]

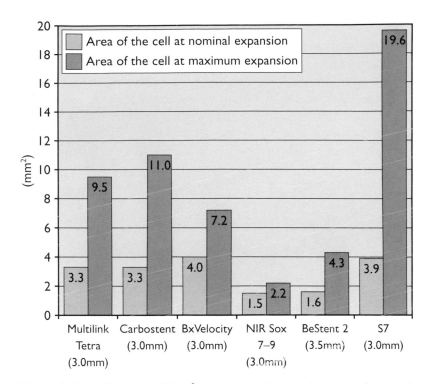

Figure 8 *Area of the stent cell (mm^2) at nominal and maximal expansion for several slotted tube stents.*

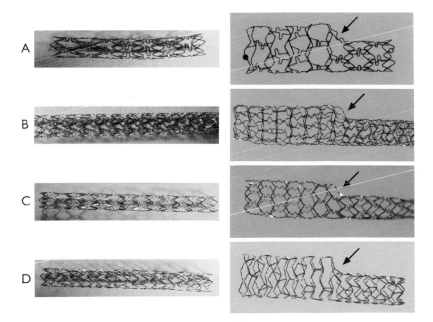

Figure 9 *Examples of stent strut prolapse from the main branch toward the side branch following kissing balloon inflation (arrows). A, The Sorin Sirius Carbostent (Sorin Biomedica Cardio, Saluggia, Italy); B, the BeStent 2 (Medtronic AVE, Minneapolis, MN); C, the BX Velocity (Cordis, a J&J Company, Warren, NJ); D, the Multi-Link Tetra stent (Guidant, Temecula, CA).*

- If a significant dissection occurs in the side branch, cross over to the decision to perform T or V stenting (see below).
- Remove the wire from the side branch and park the wire in the proximal segment of the main vessel that will not be covered by the stent.
- Position the stent in the main branch and expand the stent at its nominal pressure, usually not more then 8atm, even if the stent is not fully expanded in its central part. It is important that the stent is fully deployed at the extremities.
- Advance the stent delivery balloon distal to the stent and cross with the original side branch wire back into the side branch. Sometimes it may be easier to remove the stent deploying the balloon from the guiding catheter and re-advance the balloon following wire crossing into the side branch.
- Advance a balloon toward the side branch without necessarily crossing into the side branch, just make sure that the tip of the balloon is well engaged into the stent, which confirms that the wire that re-crossed into the side branch is not under the stent struts. The balloon may not cross into the side branch, because the struts of the stent may not be fully open
- Pull back the stent delivery balloon into the stent and perform a high-pressure inflation (12–16atm).
- Advance the balloon into the side branch and perform an inflation sufficient to fully expand the balloon.
- Perform a final kissing inflation at moderate pressure (6–8atm).

If the operator considers it appropriate to stent both branches, we recommend the modified T or V techniques.

The modified 'T' stent technique

This technique with kissing stents can be employed when the side branch originates with an angle of 90° or close to 90° [20,21] (Figure 10). Both branches are wired and alternately dilated. A first stent is advanced into the side branch but not expanded and a second stent is advanced in the main branch, covering the ostium of the side branch. Then, the first stent is carefully positioned at the ostium of the side branch and expanded, followed by the removal of the balloon and wire from the side branch. Then the stent in the main branch is expanded, the side branch is rewired, and kissing balloon dilatations of both branches are performed.

This technique is very safe, as both stents are positioned before inflation, abolishing the difficulties in crossing a second stent. It allows exact positioning of the first stent at the ostium of the side branch. In case of slight protrusion of the first stent into the main branch while dilating the second stent, the first stent might be pushed into the side branch.

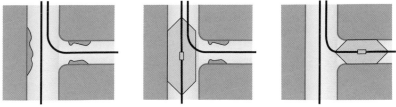

1: Wire and dilate both branches.

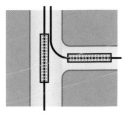

2: Positioning of both unexpanded stents.

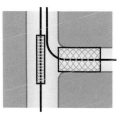

3: Dilatation of the stent at the ostium of the side branch.

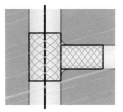

4: Removal of wire and balloon from side branch and dilatation of stent in main

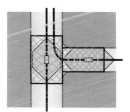

5: Rewiring of the side branch and final kissing balloon dilatation.

Figure 10 *Scheme of the 'modified T' stent technique.*

Disadvantages of this procedure are that it is limited to close to 90° bifurcations, and that if the stent in the side branch is implanted too distal, an uncovered gap might remain at the ostium of the side branch.

A final kissing inflation may not be necessary if the result appears adequate.

When we perform this technique, we prefer a ring type of stent of the S family (Medtronic AVE, Minneapolis, MN) for the side branch. For the main branch the ideal stent should one with a very open cell design, such as the BiodivYsio OC or an S670.

The reason why we recommend a ring stent for the side branch is that, in case the stent initially protrudes into the main branch, it is possible to slightly push the stent strut toward the side branch without causing a rupture of the balloon which is deploying the stent in the main branch.

The 'V' stent technique

This is a kissing stents technique suitable for bifurcations of two large side branches with a large diameter of the vessel proximal to the bifurcation. As the names implies, this technique is best suited for branches that originate with a narrow angle (less than 70°, Figure 11). Again, both branches are wired and alternately predilated. Subsequently, the two unexpanded stents are positioned close to the ostium of the branches with a slight abutment into the main vessel. It is better to expand the two stents alternately to avoid dislodgment of one balloon during simultaneous inflations. High-pressure inflation with, eventually, short balloons might be performed alternately, but the final inflation should be simultaneous ('kissing') using the same pressure and appropriately sized balloons.

> Using this technique a metallic neocarina is created within the vessel proximal to the bifurcation.

Theoretical concerns about this carina as regards an increased risk of thrombosis have not been confirmed in our experience. The most

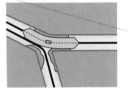

Both branches are wired and dilated

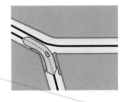

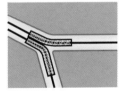

a) Positioning of two parallel stents covering the main vessel proximal to the bifurcation and both branches.

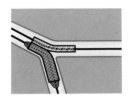

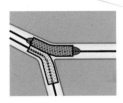

b) Inflation of first one and then the second stent (alternate dilatation).

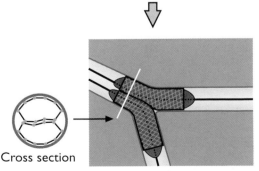

Cross section

Final kissing balloon inflation using same pressure for both balloons.

Figure 11 *Scheme of the 'V' stent technique.*

appropriate stents for this technique are two slotted tube stents of equal design with good radial strength to preserve the best configuration of the proximal carina. This technique is safe, since access to both branches is always maintained. The lesion coverage is also complete. The quick performance, the easy execution, and the safety are the major advantages of the 'V' technique.

Intravascular ultrasound (IVUS) guidance is important in this situation to check that both stents are well expanded at their proximal ends.

> We performed several implantations with this technique, and the creation of a proximal carina did not lead to stent thrombosis.

The culotte technique is another approach to be considered when the angle between the two branches is acute.

Particular techniques

An interesting new approach in treating bifurcational lesions is the use of debulking with rotational atherectomy, directional atherectomy (when possible)[22] or, more recently, the cutting balloon before stent implantation. It remains to be determined if the reduction in restenosis is sufficient to justify the complexity and the cost of the procedure.

It is clear that debulking prior to stenting is essential when the predilating balloon does not fully expand. In this event, we favor rotational atherectomy or the cutting balloon.

Lesions located at the left main stem

Percutaneous treatment of left main stem lesions is currently performed on a protected left main stem or on selected patients without protected circulation.[23-26] The clinical indications for treating these lesions with stent implantation are not discussed here: we discuss only the technical aspects involved in stent selection.

Treatment of left main stems lesions involves treatment of an aorto-ostial lesion and/or of a lesion located in the body of the left main stem. In a few situations there is the need to treat the distal left main as a bifurcational lesion.

The size of the left main artery is quite favorable to stent implantation in terms of restenosis rate. The major problem is that in an unprotected left main artery, stent restenosis may manifest either with sudden death or with unstable angina, rapidly followed by death.

> For this reason, when stent implantation in an unprotected left main artery is clinically indicated, most of the time we debulk the lesion with directional atherectomy to minimize the risk of restenosis.

For a discussion on stent selection, see the earlier sections on ostial lesions and bifurcational lesions. The only unique aspect of left main stem stenting is the final size of this vessel. It is not unusual, especially if IVUS is employed, to perform a stent postdilatation with a balloon over 4mm. For this reason, when the left main artery appears large, we recommend usage of slotted tubular stents that can be expanded over 4mm diameter. The NIR 9-cell, the BX Velocity, the Tetra, or the Ultra are excellent choices.

> When the stent is overexpanded, it is important to take into account that a significant foreshortening will occur. If the stent is being deployed to treat an aorto-ostial lesion, stent foreshortening can leave the ostium uncovered.

The operator should be aware of this fact when initially placing the stent, and he should not hesitate to place a second stent in case the ostium is left uncovered. The usage of stents with no foreshortening and with markers like those of the BeStent or the Carbostent is an important consideration to keep in mind. As a general rule, when treating an aorto-ostial lesion it is important to avoid using a stent which is very short, such as an 8 or 9mm stent. This recommendation becomes even more important when dealing with a lesion at the ostium of the left main artery. It is not rare to see a stent that becomes ejected from the left main stem at the time of postdilatation owing to its short anchoring length.

Calcified lesions

Despite the widespread notion that calcium affects stent expansion,[27] few reports specifically deal with this issue.[28,29] The general view is that stent expansion in a calcified lesion will yield a smaller final lumen than will expansion in a noncalcified lesion. Adequate final expansion is usually achieved by stretching the softer part of the wall. If an adequate final lumen is achieved, this approach does not seem to affect restenosis. To obtain a good final lumen size, it is important to have a slotted tubular stent with minimal recoil and good radial strength. This requirement is needed because frequently the lumen gain occurs by stretching the noncalcified arc of the vessel.

> The NIR stent, the Bx Velocity, the Tetra, or the stents of the S family are all reasonable choices.

The operator should not forget that in calcified lesions the preparation of the lesion for stent implantation is the more important part of the procedure and that the amount of calcium visible on X-ray does not correlate with the amount of calcium on IVUS and, more importantly, with the superficial or deep location.[30]

Every effort to evaluate the lesion and to prepare the lesion with rotational atherectomy or with cutting balloon will be well rewarded.

A post dilatation with a short noncompliant balloon is another important step. The operator should remember the importance of achieving an immediate optimal result by lesion preparation and stent postdilation and the importance of keeping the result by utilizing a stent with minimal recoil.

Chronic total occlusions

Stent implantation for chronic total occlusions has to deal with two problems: (1) the amount of plaque mass in these types of lesions is large, and (2) it is not rare that the passage through the occluded segment occurs by creating a false lumen with reentry.

These two elements mandate the insertion of a stent with good lesion coverage and radial support. The Palmaz–Schatz stent was the one used in the Stenting In Chronic Coronary Occlusion (SICCO) study,[31] which reported significant benefits of stent implantation (32% restenosis) in comparison with PTCA (74% restenosis) after recanalization of chronic total occlusions. In the Total Occlusion Study of Canada (TOSCA),[32] 410 patients with nonacute native coronary occlusions were randomized to percutaneous transluminal coronary angioplasty (PTCA) or primary stenting with the heparin-coated Palmaz–Schatz stent. With 95.6% angiographic follow-up, primary stenting resulted in a 44% reduction in failed patency (10.9% versus 19.5%, P = 0.024) and a 45% reduction in clinically driven target-vessel revascularization at 6 months (15.4% versus 8.4%, P = 0.03).

In addition to various slotted tubular stents (NIR, Bx Velocity), the Wallstent needs to be considered for dealing with a large vessel, especially for the right coronary artery.[33]

The general concept to be followed is to use a stent with good plaque coverage, such as the slotted tubular stents with a closed cell design.

Vessels smaller than 3.0mm in diameter

Stent implantation in small vessels is accompanied by a number of problems. First, no stents were specifically made to be expanded in small vessels with the capacity to gain optimal radial support at diameters between 2.5 and 3mm. Only recently have stents such as the Mini Crown, the BeStent (4 crowns), the BiodivYsio SV (Small Vessels), the 6-cell Bx Velocity, the Multi-Link Pixel stent, the 2.5mm 4-cell Carbostent and the small-vessel PURA Vario AS, which are designed to fit vessels below 3mm, become available. The most important attributes of these stents are their good flexibility, their capacity to reach quite distal lesions, and the very thin strut structure of most of them.

> One particular feature of our experience of implanting stents in vessels with angiographic diameter less than 3mm is that the balloon:artery ratio for the final stent dilatation is significantly higher than the ratio employed in larger vessels (1.29 for small vessels versus. 1.09 for larger vessels; p <0.0001).

The explanation for this choice is that we use the information obtained by IVUS to maximize the lumen gain, particularly in small vessels. The amount of plaque (which decreases the angiographic lumen size) and the arterial remodeling (which enlarges the vessel size, as measured by IVUS) explain the differences between angiographic balloon sizing in comparison with balloon sizing by IVUS. In some situations the vessel size measured by IVUS as media-to-media diameter can be 1mm larger than the lumen diameter measured by quantitative coronary angiography (QCA) (Figure 12). At follow-up, the higher restenosis rate seen in small vessels was associated with a loss index that was significantly higher than that obtained in large vessels (0.56 vs. 0.45; p = 0.0006).[34] We can only speculate on the possible causes for this higher loss index. Hypotheses include wall trauma resulting from aggressive dilatation, the use of stents not perfectly suited to be implanted on vessels smaller than 3mm (higher recoil, more metal in relation to the vessel surface area), or a combination of the two. As demonstrated by Moussa et al.,[35] it is possible that in small vessels the relationship between final lumen diameter or IVUS cross-sectional area and angiographic restenosis may not be linear (Figure 13).

The recent introduction of stents specifically designed for small vessels has allowed the performance of randomized trials with no noise coming from the implantation of stents not dedicated to small vessels. Figure 14 summarizes the results of four recently completed studies.[36–39] In three of the studies the BeStent 4 crowns (Medtronic AVE, Minneapolis, MN) was used; in the other study the Multi-Link was initially implanted and then substituted by the Duet (Guidant, Temecula, CA).

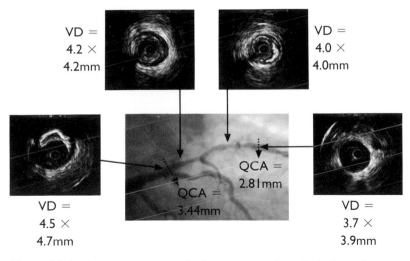

Figure 12 *Difference between quantitative coronary angiography (QCA) and intravascular ultrasound (IVUS) in measurement of reference vessel diameter. VD = vessel diameter.*

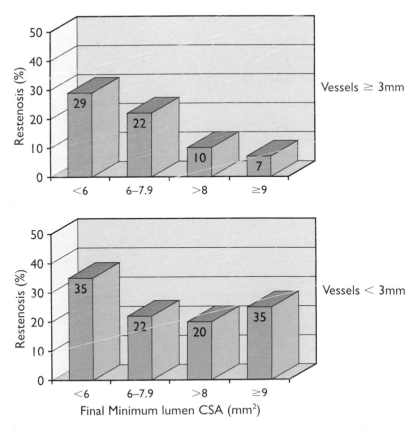

Figure 13 *Restenosis rates according to final minimal lumen cross-sectional area (CSA) and reference vessel size.*

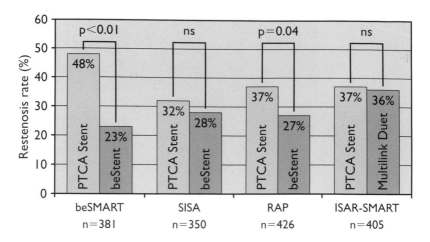

Figure 14 *Restenosis rates in randomized trials of small vessel stenting versus balloon angioplasty (PTCA); BESMART = BeStent in SMall ARTeries; SISA = Stenting In Small Arteries; RAP = Restenosis en Arterias Pequenas; ISAR-SMART = Intracoronary Stenting or Angioplasty for Restenosis reduction in SMall ARTeries; n = number of patients enrolled.*

The results showed a superiority of the stent versus PTCA in two studies and equivalence in the other two.

An interesting and important observation came from the subanalysis of the ISAR study, named ISAR-STEREO.[40] The authors reported a significantly lower restenosis rate in vessels larger than 2.8mm (15.0% versus. 25.8%, p <0.003) at follow-up following the implantation of the thin-strut (0.05mm) Multi-Link compared to the thicker Duet (0.14mm). Whether this finding also applies to small vessels needs to be evaluated.

For all these reasons, and to ensure more flexibility and easier delivery to lesions located on small vessels, we suggest implanting vessels <3mm with dedicated small vessel stents with thin struts. The BiodivYsio SV and the BeStent (4 crowns) are probably the most suitable stents to be implanted in lesions located in small vessels. The delivery system of these stents is about 0.75 mm in profile, making them the smallest profile stent delivery system. The Sorin Carbostent is another thin-strut stent available in a small vessel size. All these stents, with the exception of the BiodivYsio SV stents, are visible under X-ray because of distal and proximal radiopaque markers.

The Bx Velocity with the dedicated 6-cell stent and the Multi-Link Pixel, a new small vessel stent by Guidant, are also good choices. In comparison with the other small vessel stents, these two stents do not belong to the family of thin-strut stents and they are visible under X-ray.

Saphenous vein grafts

Implanting stents in lesions in saphenous vein grafts usually involves dealing with a lesion located on a large vessel. The goals of minimizing trauma to the plaque and giving maximum lesion coverage to avoid the risk of distal embolization bring the self-expandable stents back into the picture. This is why we consider the Wallstent to be the most suitable device for lesions in these locations, despite unsatisfactory early results: a 7.6% rate of mortality and a 24% rate of complete occlusion reported in 1991.[41,42]

The results subsequently improved, with a decrease in the incidence of stent occlusion (3.4%), but there remained a high incidence of hemorrhagic complications (17%).[43] During the following years results improved, mainly because of increased experience,[44] better deployment techniques, and the introduction of a combined antiplatelet regimen.

One persisting problem with stent implantation in vein grafts is that future events may result from progression of other lesions that were not considered critical at the time of initial stent implantation on the target lesion.[45] This issue will be evaluated by prospective studies comparing a strategy of focal stent implantation on the critical lesions with a strategy aimed at stenting, and also implanting stents in lesions not angiographically critical.

> For all these reasons, vein graft stent implantation must be performed with a stent with optimal lesion coverage and available in different lengths (vein grafts require longer stents).

The Wallstent best satisfies these requirements. For more focal lesions, the Ultra version of the Multi-Link design specifically made for vein graft lesions (Guidant, Temecula, CA), and the 9-cell NIR stent are good choices.

The other issue unique to vein grafts is the risk of distal embolization. It has been our experience that no particular stent currently available is more likely than another to limit these complications. The recent introduction of a protective balloon on a wire system (the SAFE[46,47] and the SAFER study -- http://www.tctmd.com/clinical-trials/breaking/one.html? presentation id=41) and of a number of filter devices has improved the safety of vein graft interventions.

Vein graft stenting will not be complete without mention of the PTFE-covered stent. This device may have the potential to better entrap the degenerated material present in vein graft, with a possible positive impact on distal embolization and late restenosis.[48,49] A similar device with the covering membrane made of bovine pericardium is currently under clinical evaluation (Figure 15).

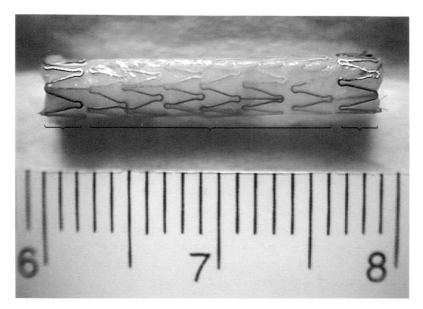

Figure 15 *A stent with the covering membrane made of bovine pericardium.*

Acute closure and threatened closure

Acute closure is the typical situation in which stents were originally applied.[50,51] The stents used most extensively are the Gianturco–Roubin I stent[52,53] and the Palmaz–Schatz stent.[54] Higher rates of success, even in complex anatomy and long dissections, have been reported with the Gianturco–Roubin II stent [55] and with the AVE II MicroStent.[56]

> We think that the ideal stent for treating a dissection with impending closure should have an easy and predictable delivery, even without an optimal guiding catheter or guidewire support.

We like to call this stent 'the panic stent.' The Tetra or the S660 (2.5mm diameter, 8mm–9mm long) is one of the most deliverable stents in complex anatomies.

Treatment of dissections may include placing a short stent distally to an already deployed stent, usually to treat a residual distal dissection not evident at the time of the first stent implantation.

> The possibility of completely sealing a dissection, especially in the setting of impending closure, remains one important predictor of stent occlusion even with the use of high-pressure dilatation after stent implantation and with administration of aspirin and ticlopidine.[57]

Therefore, the stent with the best predictable delivery and about which the operator feels confident is likely to be the preferred one: it will also be the one with the lowest incidence of stent thrombosis if it provides good dissection coverage (no prolapse) and has been implanted correctly.

Special situations

There are conditions in which the operator needs to modify the tools available in order to provide a new device capable of satisfying a need. Three of these conditions are the treatment of severe focal aneurysmal dilatation of the coronary arteries, the treatment of more diffuse aneurysmal disease of vein grafts, and, occasionally, the treatment of coronary perforations. The use of an autologous vein graft-coated stent is an interesting solution pioneered by Stefanadis and associates.[58,59] The Tetra stent, the Bx Velocity, or the NIR stent and other slotted tubular stents are good platforms on which the autologous vein can be mounted. Coronary perforations are rare but need rapid and effective treatment.

> The new PTFE-covered stent now available premounted is probably the best device to use to treat a coronary perforation[60] or to treat a coronary aneurysm.[61,62]

Conclusions

Among all the theoretical and practical considerations and reasons we give for selecting a particular stent to treat a specific lesion, the experience and confidence of the operator should stay at the top of the list.

No rationale for choosing a specific stent for a specific lesion is yet supported by randomized trials. Nonetheless, a large number of observational studies support the view expressed in this chapter.

> Except for bailout stent implantation, stents are implanted with the intention of preventing restenosis; therefore, the operator should strive to reach this goal within the framework of patient safety.

Optimal stent selection, balloon sizing, and lesion preparation, when necessary, to achieve an optimal result in terms of final lumen dimensions remain the most important goals in percutaneous coronary interventions.

References

1. Serruys PW, de Jaegere P, Kiemeneij F et al. A comparison of balloon-expandable-stent implantation with balloon angioplasty in patients with coronary artery disease. BENESTENT Study Group. N Engl J Med 1994;331:489–95.
2. Fischman DL, Leon MB, Baim DS et al. A randomized comparison of coronary-stent placement and balloon angioplasty in the treatment of coronary artery disease. Stent Restenosis Study Investigators. N Engl J Med 1994;331:496–501.
3. Colombo A, Hall P, Nakamura S et al. Intracoronary stenting without anticoagulation accomplished with intravascular ultrasound guidance. Circulation 1995;91:1676–88.
4. Karrillon GJ, Morice MC, Benveniste E et al. Intracoronary stent implantation without ultrasound guidance and with replacement of conventional anticoagulation by antiplatelet therapy. 30-day clinical outcome of the French Multicenter Registry. Circulation 1996;94:1519–27.
5. Schomig A, Neumann FJ, Kastrati A et al. A randomized comparison of antiplatelet and anticoagulant therapy after the placement of coronary-artery stents. N Engl J Med 1996;334:1084–9.
6. Kuntz RE, Safian RD, Carrozza JP, Fishman RF, Mansour M, Baim DS. The importance of acute luminal diameter in determining restenosis after coronary atherectomy or stenting. Circulation 1992;86:1827–35.
7. Zidar JP, Fry E, Lambert C et al. The Venus Trial: a multicenter registry of the Cordis Bx Velocity stent. Am J Cardiol 2000;86:17i-38.
8. Sousa JE, Costa MA, Abizaid A et al. Lack of neointimal proliferation after implantation of sirolimus-coated stents in human coronary arteries: a quantitative coronary angiography and three-dimensional intravascular ultrasound study. Circulation 2001;103:192–5.
9. Wentzel JJ, Krams R, Schuurbiers JC et al. Relationship between neointimal thickness and shear stress after Wallstent implantation in human coronary arteries. Circulation 2001;103:1740–5.
10. Baim DS, Cutlip DE, O'Shaughnessy CD et al. Final results of a randomized trial comparing the NIR stent to the Palmaz–Schatz stent for narrowings in native coronary arteries. Am J Cardiol 2001;87:152–6.
11. Phillips PS, Alfonso F, Segovia J et al. Effects of Palmaz–Schatz stents on angled coronary arteries. Am J Cardiol 1997;79:191–3.
12. Antoniucci D, Bartorelli A, Valenti R et al. Clinical and angiographic outcome after coronary arterial stenting with the carbostent. Am J Cardiol 2000;85:821–5.
13. Koster R, Vieluf D, Kiehn M et al. Nickel and molybdenum contact allergies in patients with coronary in-stent restenosis. Lancet 2000;356:1895–7.
14. Zampieri P, Colombo A, Almagor Y, Maiello L, Finci L. Results of coronary stenting of ostial lesions. Am J Cardiol 1994;73:901–3.
15. Kerwin PM, McKeever LS, Marek JC, Hartmann JR, Enger EL. Directional atherectomy of aorto-ostial stenoses. Cathet Cardiovasc Diagn 1993;Suppl:17–25.
16. Stephan WJ, Bates ER, Garratt KN, Hinohara T, Muller DW. Directional atherectomy of coronary and saphenous vein graft ostial stenoses. Am J Cardiol 1995;75:1015–18.
17. Kastrati A, Schomig A, Dirschinger J et al. Increased risk of restenosis after placement of gold-coated stents: results of a randomized trial comparing gold-coated with uncoated steel stents in patients with coronary artery disease. Circulation 2000;101:2478–83.

18. Yamashita T, Nishida T, Adamian MG et al. Bifurcation lesions: two stents versus one stent – immediate and follow-up results. J Am Coll Cardiol 2000;35:1145–51.

19. Ormiston J, Webster M, Ruygrok P, Scot D, Stewart J. Stent distortion during simulated side-branch dilatation. J Am Coll Cardiol 1998;31:18A.

20. Nakamura S, Hall P, Maiello L, Colombo A. Techniques for Palmaz–Schatz stent deployment in lesions with a large side branch. Cathet Cardiovasc Diagn 1995;34:353–61.

21. Carrie D, Karouny E, Chouairi S, Puel J. "T"-shaped stent placement: a technique for the treatment of dissected bifurcation lesions. Cathet Cardiovasc Diagn 1996;37:311–13.

22. Karvouni E, Di Mario C, Nishida T et al. Directional atherectomy prior to stenting in bifurcation lesions: a matched comparison study with stenting alone. Cathet Cardiovasc Intervent 2001;52: in press.

23. Black AJ, Cortina R, Bossi I, Choussat R, Fajadet J, Marco J. Unprotected left main coronary artery stenting: correlates of midterm survival and impact of patient selection. J Am Coll Cardiol 2001;37:832–8.

24. Silvestri M, Barragan P, Sainsous J et al. Unprotected left main coronary artery stenting: immediate and medium-term outcomes of 140 elective procedures. J Am Coll Cardiol 2000;35:1543–50.

25. Park SJ, Park SW, Hong MK et al. Stenting of unprotected left main coronary artery stenoses: immediate and late outcomes. J Am Coll Cardiol 1998;31:37–42.

26. Ellis SG, Tamai H, Nobuyoshi M et al. Contemporary percutaneous treatment of unprotected left main coronary stenoses: initial results from a multicenter registry analysis 1994–1996. Circulation 1997;96:3867–72.

27. Hodgson JM. Oh no, even stenting is affected by calcium! Cathet Cardiovasc Diagn 1996;38:236–7.

28. Albrecht D, Kaspers S, Fussl R, Hopp HW, Sechtem U. Coronary plaque morphology affects stent deployment: assessment by intracoronary ultrasound. Cathet Cardiovasc Diagn 1996;38:229–35.

29. Moussa I, Di Mario C, Moses J et al. Coronary stenting after rotational atherectomy in calcified and complex lesions. Angiographic and clinical follow-up results. Circulation 1997;96:128-

30. Mintz GS, Popma JJ, Pichard AD et al. Patterns of calcification in coronary artery disease. A statistical analysis of intravascular ultrasound and coronary angiography in 1155 lesions. Circulation 1995;91:1959–65.

31. Sirnes PA, Golf S, Myreng Y et al. Stenting in Chronic Coronary Occlusion (SICCO): a randomized, controlled trial of adding stent implantation after successful angioplasty. J Am Coll Cardiol 1996;28:1444–51.

32. Buller CE, Dzavik V, Carere RG et al. Primary stenting versus balloon angioplasty in occluded coronary arteries: the Total Occlusion Study of Canada (TOSCA). Circulation 1999;100:236–42.

33. Ozaki Y, Violaris AG, Hamburger J et al. Short- and long-term clinical and quantitative angiographic results with the new, less shortening Wallstent for vessel reconstruction in chronic total occlusion: a quantitative angiographic study. J Am Coll Cardiol 1996;28:354–60.

34. Akiyama T, Moussa I, Reimers B et al. Angiographic and clinical outcome following coronary stenting of small vessels: a comparison with coronary stenting of large vessels. J Am Coll Cardiol 1998;32:1610–18.

35. Moussa I, Moses J, Wang X, Colombo A. Does "the bigger is better" hypothesis after coronary stenting apply in small vessels. J Am Coll Cardiol 1998;31:1060–87.

36. Garcia E G-RM, Pasalodos J, Bethancourt A, Zueco J, Iniguez A. Immediate

results of the RAP study: a randomized trial that compares stents and balloon angioplasty in small vessels. Eur Heart J 1999;20:385.

37. Schalij M DS, Reiber JHC, Bilodeau L, van Weert A. The stenting in small artries study (SISA): 6 months quantitative angiographic results. Eur Heart J 2000;21:262.

38. Kleiman NS CR. Results from late-breaking clinical trials session at ACCIS 2000 and ACC 2000. J Am Coll Cardiol 2000;36:310–25.

39. Kastrati A, Dischinger J, Mehilli J et al. Intracoronary stenting or angioplasty for restenosis reduction in small-arteries (ISAR-SMART) trial. Eur Heart J 2000;21:262.

40. Kastrati A, Mehilli J, Dirschinger J et al. Intracoronary stenting and angiographic results: strut thickness effect on restenosis outcome (ISAR-STEREO) trial. Circulation 2001;103:2816–21.

41. Serruys PW, Strauss BH, Beatt KJ et al. Angiographic follow-up after placement of a self-expanding coronary-artery stent. N Engl J Med 1991;324:13–17.

42. de Scheerder IK, Strauss BH, de Feyter PJ et al. Stenting of venous bypass grafts: a new treatment modality for patients who are poor candidates for reintervention. Am Heart J 1992;123:1046–54.

43. Keane D, Buis B, Reifart N et al. Clinical and angiographic outcome following implantation of the new Less Shortening Wallstent in aortocoronary vein grafts: introduction of a second generation stent in the clinical arena. J Intervent Cardiol 1994;7:557–64.

44. de Jaegere PP, van Domburg RT, Feyter PJ et al. Long-term clinical outcome after stent implantation in saphenous vein grafts. J Am Coll Cardiol 1996;28:89–96.

45. Hartmann JR, McKeever LS, O'Neill WW et al. Recanalization of chronically occluded aortocoronary saphenous vein bypass grafts with long-term, low dose direct infusion of urokinase (ROBUST): a serial trial. J Am Coll Cardiol 1996;27:60–6.

46. Grube E, Webb J, Prpic R et al. Clinical safety and efficacy of the PercuSurge guidewire in the saphenous vein graft angioplasty free of emboli (SAFE) study. J Am Coll Cardiol 2000;35:41.

47. Gerckens U, Muller R, Rowold S, Grube E. The Filterwire (tm): first evaluation of a new protection catheter device for distal embolization in native coronary arteries in SVGs. J Am Coll Cardiol 2001;37:1A–648A.

48. Briguori C, De Gregorio J, Nishida T et al. Polytetrafluoroethylene-covered stent for the treatment of narrowings in aorticocoronary saphenous vein grafts. Am J Cardiol 2000;86:343–6.

49. Baldus S, Koster R, Elsner M et al. Treatment of aortocoronary vein graft lesions with membrane-covered stents: a multicenter surveillance trial. Circulation 2000;102:2024–7.

50. Herrmann HC, Buchbinder M, Clemen MW et al. Emergent use of balloon-expandable coronary artery stenting for failed percutaneous transluminal coronary angioplasty. Circulation 1992;86:812–19.

51. Roubin GS, Cannon AD, Agrawal SK et al. Intracoronary stenting for acute and threatened closure complicating percutaneous transluminal coronary angioplasty. Circulation 1992;85:916–27.

52. George BS, Voorhees WD, 3rd, Roubin GS et al. Multicenter investigation of coronary stenting to treat acute or threatened closure after percutaneous transluminal coronary angioplasty: clinical and angiographic outcomes. J Am Coll Cardiol 1993;22:135–43.

53. Sutton JM, Ellis SG, Roubin GS et al. Major clinical events after coronary stenting. The multicenter registry of acute and elective Gianturco–Roubin

stent placement. The Gianturco–Roubin Intracoronary Stent Investigator Group. Circulation 1994;89:1126–37.

54. Schomig A, Kastrati A, Mudra H et al. Four-year experience with Palmaz–Schatz stenting in coronary angioplasty complicated by dissection with threatened or present vessel closure. Circulation 1994;90:2716–24.

55. Leon MB, Fry E, O'Shaughnessy CD. Preliminary multicenter experiences with the new GR-II stent for abrupt and threatened closure syndrome. Circulation. 1996;94:I–207.

56. Ozaki Y, Keane D, Ruygrok P, de Feyter P, Stertzer S, Serruys PW. Acute clinical and angiographic results with the new AVE Micro coronary stent in bailout management. Am J Cardiol 1995;76:112–16.

57. Moussa I, Di Mario C, Reimers B, Akiyama T, Tobis J, Colombo A. Subacute stent thrombosis in the era of intravascular ultrasound-guided coronary stenting without anticoagulation: frequency, predictors and clinical outcome. J Am Coll Cardiol 1997;29:6–12.

58. Stefanadis C, Toutouzas P. Percutaneous implantation of autologous vein graft stent for treatment of coronary artery disease. Lancet 1995;345:1509.

59. Stefanadis C, Toutouzas K, Vlachopoulos C et al. Autologous vein graft-coated stent for treatment of coronary artery disease. Cathet Cardiovasc Diagn 1996;38:159–70.

60. Briguori C, Nishida T, Anzuini A, Di Mario C, Grube E, Colombo A. Emergency polytetrafluoroethylene-covered stent implantation to treat coronary ruptures. Circulation 2000;102:3028–31.

61. Di Mario C, Inglese L, Colombo A. Treatment of a coronary aneurysm with a new polytetrafluoethylene-coated stent: a case report. Catheter Cardiovasc Intervent 1999;46:463–5.

62. Heuser RR, Woodfield S, Lopez A. Obliteration of a coronary artery aneurysm with a PTFE-covered stent: endoluminal graft for coronary disease revisited. Catheter Cardiovasc Intervent 1999;46:113–16.